CORTISOL

THE MASTER HORMONE

CORTISOL
THE MASTER HORMONE

Improve Your Health, Weight, Fertility, Menopause, Longevity, and Reduce Stress

Wibe Wagemans
Ioana Bina MD PhD FACG

CORTISOL: The Master Hormone
By Wibe Wagemans & Ioana Bina, MD PhD FACG

Copyright © 2022 by Pardigm Inc.

Published by
Pardigm Inc.
541 Jefferson Ave, Suite 100
Redwood City, CA 94063

All rights reserved. No part of this book may be reproduced in whole or in part without written permission from the publisher, except by reviewers who may quote brief excerpts in connection with a review in a newspaper, magazine, or electronic publication; nor may any part of this book be reproduced, stored in a retrieval system, or transmitted in any form or by any means electronic, mechanical, photocopying, recording, or other, without written permission from the publisher.

Print ISBN: 979-8-9861680-2-9

Printed in the United States of America

CONTENTS

Legal Disclaimer	vi
An Invitation	vii
Foreword	xiii
1. Get to Know Us Because We Want to Know You	1
2. Why You Should Measure Your Cortisol Levels	14
3. How Monitoring Cortisol Can Help Manage Burnout, Stress and Mental Disorders	33
4. Why Elite Athletes Measure Their Cortisol	43
5. Stress, Infertility, and Cortisol	55
6. Stress, Menopause, and Cortisol	66
7. What's the Gut and the Microbiome Got to Do with Cortisol?	74
8. Cortisol and Weight Loss: Why So Many Diets Fail	84
9. Cortisol for The Diagnosis of Long Covid?	96
10. Scientific Breakthrough: Mindset Controls Cortisol	100
11. Recommendations: How to Keep Your Cortisol Levels Balanced	108
For More Information	137
Erratum	138
Pardigm.com intro	139
Notes	141

Legal Disclaimer

This book is intended to provide helpful and informative material, including the opinions and conclusions of the authors with respect to some vitally important medical issues. On some medical issues, there is consensus among scientists, and on others, scientists do not agree (yet). This book is not intended to replace the advice of a physician. Nothing in this book is intended to replace guideline recommendations or promote specific therapies for individual cases. Always consult your physician or qualified healthcare professional on any matters regarding your health before adopting any suggestions in this book, or drawing inferences from it. The authors and publishers specifically disclaim any liability, loss, or risk, personal or otherwise, that is incurred as a consequence, directly or indirectly, of the use and application of any of the contents, or in the promotion of this book.

An Invitation

Did you know that out-of-balance cortisol is often the No. 1 or No. 2 cause of:

- Infertility
- Menopause symptoms
- Athletic readiness
- Weight gain
- Insulin resistance
- Burnout
- Depression
- Insomnia
- Cardiovascular disease
- Early death

Say hello to cortisol, your body's master hormone.

It's the friend that helped your ancestors flee predators in the African savannas. It's the enemy, though, when it overreacts and hangs around too long – damaging every cell and biological process in your body.

Cortisol is the body's alarm system that makes your heart pound when you parachute out of an airplane or sit down to take a college entrance exam. It tells you to *act now* to save your life. But it can also send you into a panic over the stresses of everyday life: Abusive workplaces, job losses, money worries, and strained relationships to name a few.

A crucial biomarker indicating the brain's response to psychological or physiological imbalances in the body, cortisol has been around millions of years before the appearance of homo sapiens.[1] Yet, medical researchers did not properly name it until

1950. It took archeologists until 2009 to detect it in the hair of Peruvians, circa 550 C.E.[2] At the very least, the presence of cortisol in nearly every part of the body, including blood, saliva, urine, cerebrospinal fluid, nails and hair, suggests that these ancient Peruvians experienced stress in their final hours.[3]

We moderns, living in a time of social media pressures, political brinkmanship, echo chambers, climate change, pandemic anxiety, and a 24/7 news cycle, have more opportunities for prolonged stress than our pre-industrial forebears.

We're here to help you manage your cortisol rhythm, so that your cortisol rhythm does not manage you. We'll do that by sharing the expertise of the world's most influential scientists with you.

We, the authors of *Cortisol: The Master Hormone*, are a serial entrepreneur and an integrative physician, and we've come together to help you make cortisol work in your favor. In practical terms, we're talking about a radically new way of measuring cortisol so you get a nuanced, real-time picture of what it's doing inside your body and mind.

Overstatement? Not at all. Here's why.

We've come up with a simple way to read your cortisol rhythm on your smartphone. Knowing when it's too high or too low can make the difference between feeling great or flubbing your performance at a board meeting, experiencing infertility issues, or having trouble losing weight. Simply by measuring cortisol with your phone – without any other device or lab – you can take charge of your health.

Measuring your cortisol is as close to a healthcare silver bullet as you can get.

Until now, checking cortisol in real time was practically impossible. You saw a doctor to get a blood, saliva or a 24-hour urine test. The sample was sent to a lab and underwent analysis. Days or weeks later, you received a result that typically gave you a single data point. Getting only one measurement is like measuring your heartbeat for one second. Our cortisol varies widely throughout the day and has a circadian – or waking/sleeping – pattern with broad health implications. To appreciate the powerful role cortisol plays, we need a more nuanced, more comprehensive picture of its behavior in the body *throughout the day*.

The app we created uses your phone's camera, which has a higher quality sensor than the average lab scanner. You'll get results as precise as those from an overnight lab. Plus, you get your results in real time – this will be available soon.[4]

Here's what you do once you have the Pardigm app on your phone.

When you wake up, collect your saliva by using a rapid test salivary strip. Next, take a picture of the strip with your phone camera. Wait a few seconds for the app's proprietary algorithms to analyze the strip and give you your exact cortisol level between 0 - 30 ng/ml. Because cortisol levels vary throughout the day in a specific pattern, you'll do this procedure five times on Day One to establish your baseline curve.[5] Now you have a story, as it were, about your physical health, mental stress, athletic overtraining, capacity for recovery, depression, infertility, menopausal symptoms, and many other issues.

What's the value to you?

The test and the results are in *your* hands, to be shared with your doctor as you see fit. They're no longer exclusively in the hands of a medical professional.

No need any longer to guess why you feel exhausted. Why you do not perform optimally in your sport, despite your constant training. Why you're overwhelmed by feelings of depression and anxiety. Knowing the basics about the science of cortisol — and understanding its connection to your overall health — will give you the *data* you need to live your best self. You'll benefit in ways you haven't even considered.

Did you know that a stress-is-enhancing mindset can help you bring cortisol to manageable levels? We'll acquaint you with the groundbreaking work of Professor Alia Crum, a Stanford Mind and Body Lab investigator and psychologist, who has studied how mindset affects human behavior, as well as physical and mental health outcomes. From her undergraduate days as an ice hockey athlete at Harvard, Dr. Crum has been interested in the power of the mind to influence our physical state. Indeed, her findings can empower you to embrace a mindset that heals your body and lets you pursue your goals – athletic, personal and professional.

Perhaps athletes, more than anyone else, know in their very muscle and sinew the devastating effect that mental stress can have on their performance. Simone Biles, Naomi Osaka, and Usain Bolt, to name a few of our generation's superior athletes, have described wild swings in mood, energy, and self-confidence. Researchers have begun to associate these mind-body fluctuations with cortisol imbalances. We cannot help but wonder how these outstanding athletes would have benefited from a cortisol-measuring tool to get themselves back in fighting trim. Indeed, we'll tell you why some Olympic athletes already measure their cortisol every day.

Measuring cortisol is not just for athletes. You'll see what we've learned about the effect of cortisol on everyone's hormones, brain function, blood pressure, bones, gut, appetite, weight, sleep patterns, immune system, and longevity. We'll help you gain insight into the impact of cortisol on women's health, especially during the years of fertility, pregnancy, and menopause. We'll help you understand the effect of cortisol on health, particularly in regard to obesity.

By now you have already used a phone app to hail a taxi, take a photo, check the weather, text your kids or friends, learn a language, set an alarm, listen to a podcast, buy groceries, and pay for coffee. Gauging the status of your cortisol levels – and other biomarkers – should be just as easy as tapping an app for every other necessity in your life.

Come along with us and we'll tell you why, as sci-fi visionary Arthur C. Clarke might have put it, "Our sufficiently advanced technology is indistinguishable from magic."

It's mind-boggling that you've had to wait until now to measure your cortisol with your phone. No need to wait much longer for this game-changing technology. Let's go.

Foreword *By Phyllis Gardner, M.D.*

Silicon Valley is famous for sunny days, grand ambitions, and lots and lots of ideas. Some ideas, like Theranos, are spectacular failures. But some, like Calm or Twin Health, are true contributions to our health. Pardigm, the app that lets you measure cortisol in your body, is in the latter camp. It's one of those good ideas that could revolutionize how people can prevent debilitating diseases.

This is my somewhat elliptical way of alluding to my role as a whistleblower in one of Silicon Valley's most ignominious frauds. It's a funny thing gaining notoriety in the twilight of my career, simply because I spotted the fakery in a young entrepreneur when so many other wily people were taken in by her. Theranos — Elizabeth Holmes's bogus biomarker company — went down in flames because it flouted inquiry, investigation, and evidence, and because it showed reckless disregard for the Hippocratic Oath: "I will abstain from all intentional wrongdoing and harm."

The healthcare industry unquestionably has a need for testing technologies that can pinpoint discrete biological molecules, detect abnormalities, and recommend treatments. Many legitimate startups are working on biosensor technology that ordinary people can use in their own homes to improve nutrition or test for chronic diseases. To date, these technologies — Pardigm among them — wisely focus on a single biomarker whose measurement can be shared with medical professionals via smartphone. For now, ethical developers must address only one biomarker at a time. It doesn't hurt to be skeptical of empires built on sand.

FOREWORD

When you want to build out an ethical biomarker product, it sometimes helps to be a jack of all trades and a master of none. With my affinity for the steep slope of the learning curve – and a willingness to ask lots of questions – I've always loved the challenge that comes from working in an enterprise in any institutional setting with intelligent, hard-working individuals. That's why I went into medicine. When I got to Harvard Medical School, I thought, "This is where I belong." The price of entry was complex, nuanced thinking. I blossomed there. I had the same experience at Massachusetts General Hospital where I trained as an intern. For better or worse, we interns were on call by ourselves. I literally had to think on my feet. Mass General turned out to be my introduction to workplace stress, but I loved it. The lessons I learned about medical care have stayed with me in my subsequent career as a professor of medicine at Stanford University.

For all my love of science, I fell in love with the corporate world.[1] The American corporation is a crucible in which ideas either gain traction or wilt under scrutiny. To that end, I ventured into entrepreneurial startups after working in executive management at several biotech companies. I include my work at Alza Corporation as VP of research and head of the Technology Institute, my work at Essex Woodlands Venture firm as an adjunct partner, and my role in the formations of Genomics Collaborative and Skolar,[2] as some of my personal-best industry accomplishments. I rounded out my industry experience by sitting on several private and public boards of directors.

You might be tempted to look at my various endeavors as a conflict of interest. But female scientists, like me, are frequently drawn to developing healthcare solutions – practical applications of our work – by blending university and corporate research. The technologies we develop have to help people. The image of the male engineer who invents a widget, and then lets somebody else figure out a use for it, is passé. Physicians and scientists — female and male — are committed to identifying problems and coming up with solutions for them.

Wibe Wagemans and his Pardigm team belong to this latter cohort. By studying the impact of cortisol on our mind and body, Pardigm has homed in on a critically important healthcare biomarker. By measuring and managing cortisol levels, the company is poised to help millions of people live longer, healthier, and even less stressful lives. Frankly, until Pardigm, we didn't have a salivary cortisol biomarker product that could give us a trendline we could study and interpret. Moreover, we didn't have an easily affordable, precise cortisol measuring tool that lets us observe a patient's cortisol behavior many times a day — the only way you can get an accurate picture of what cortisol is doing in the body.[3] Best of all, these measurements can be done at home more cheaply than in a lab.

It shouldn't surprise me that Pardigm's current scientific advisory board consists of four MD- and PhD-level female scientists who have made it their goal to do work that demonstrably improves lives. Indeed, Ioana Bina, this book's co-author, is an esteemed colleague.

One of the western world's favorite myths is that invention happens by dumb luck: Some quaint individual tinkers in a garage or attic and comes up with a gadget. That's not how Pardigm rolls. Our team intentionally started by solving a problem right out of the gate. Being rational thinkers with a dream, we have not left our mission to chance. We've sought to develop a measuring and management tool for cortisol that one day could serve as a template to measure other biomarkers too. Our goal is to develop replicable methods and protocols. If results can't be reproduced, that unworkable product iteration goes into the scrapheap of healthcare boondoggles.

I've had a great personal and professional life. I'm proud of my career-long affiliations with universities and companies dedicated to advancing the health and knowledge of people on a grand scale. Anything of value needs an ardent defender, and I'll always defend the need for exacting due diligence. In practicing responsible healthcare, we can't afford to tolerate halfway measures. We can't afford to fake it 'til we make it. All of us in the medical and biotech community need to stand for good science and technological integrity. There's too much at stake to do anything less — and so much to gain.

Chapter 1

Get To Know Us Because We Want to Know You

Dr. Bina here. Working with Wibe is a thrill! We were introduced when he was looking for a cortisol expert with clinical experience to help with the best applications for his innovative technology. I have experienced first hand why cortisol is the Master Hormone! My patients don't have Cushing or Addison, but 80% are on a spectrum of cortisol imbalance that needs fixing. I knew immediately how great a quick and accurate salivary cortisol test would be - for clinicians, researchers, and patients alike. And my instincts were right. There hasn't been a week where we have not picked up, hot off the press, exciting research involving cortisol and its far-reaching effects. After all, in 2022, over 3700 scientific publications mention salivary cortisol. Late at night, you can often find us sharing our findings, energized by our enthusiasm, the phone-screen light, and a little extra cortisol.

My international education — a medical degree and a PhD from the Carol Davila University of Medicine and Pharmacy in Bucharest, my postgraduate research work in endocrinology, nutrition, and metabolism at the Université de Rouen, a Yale University-affiliated training in internal medicine and gastroenterology, and my ongoing education in personalized and functional medicine – makes me the ideal advocate for an integrative approach to health.

I am a strong proponent of "personalized medicine," a mode of medical care that customizes treatment for each individual. Indeed, I have synthesized my education and clinical work to come up with an approach that looks at the impact of stress on the whole human being, and that asks, "What can my patient learn about healthy living by addressing what's going on specifically with her gut, her hormones, her genetic make-up, the stresses in her life, and the toxicities in her environment? What therapies can I, the physician, offer that will create balance in her body and mind, perhaps for the first time in a long time?"

Early on in my twenty-year clinical career as a physician, I began to see the limitations of conventional medicine. There is no better system for severe acute lifesaving situations and procedures, but it falls short in dealing with complex chronic multisystem problems. I was responding to my patients' symptoms, but somehow not getting to the source of their gastroenterological problems. It was clear to me that oftentimes, barriers to healing stemmed from psychological stressors and maladaptive stress responses down to the cellular level. I had known about cortisol since medical school, but before working on this book, I didn't fully appreciate the wide gap between the diverse cortisol/stress-related research and what clinicians actually know and implement from these research findings. By speaking with colleagues and friends, and by witnessing the excellent results, I got interested in functional and integrative medicine —a systems-based approach to identifying the root cause of disease and create a personalized treatment plan. I realized that problems in the gut could be the result of various biological malfunctions also involving the endocrine, immune, and nervous systems.

Research on the gut microbiome – the trillions of microorganisms in your intestinal tract – is exploding. The impact of the microbiome on our immune system, hormones, body composition, weight, mental health, and risk for numerous diseases, to enumerate only a few, is absolutely astounding. After all, 95% of the body's serotonin – a signaling molecule that plays a key role in our mood, cognition and other bodily functions from digestion to sexual desire – is produced by the gut.[1] The gut microbiome also acts as a virtual endocrine organ,[2] regulating sex hormone levels.[3] And gut-educated, antibody-producing immune cells defend the brain.[4] We'll see in Chapter 7 how cortisol affects our gut and facilitates the communication between our brain and the gut microbiome.

My intuition that disease is multifactorial led me, ironically, to take a look at cortisol, the unique corticosteroid hormone produced by the body's adrenal glands — themselves regulated via the brain's hypothalamic-pituitary-adrenal (HPA) axis — and then released like a team of horses into the bloodstream. I never sought a theory of everything, but the more I studied cortisol, the more I saw the pervasive impact it has on virtually every system in the body and how it runs the show.

Indeed, I have concluded that cortisol is our biological legacy. As the primary end-product of the **HPA** axis' response to stress, cortisol shows us what's happening in the brain, and it affects every process in our body. Professor Angela Clow, a Westminster University researcher studying the biochemistry of stress, describes cortisol as a non-invasive window to the brain, highlighting the potential of salivary cortisol as both product and mediator of brain function, instrumental in disturbing brain health. [5] Salivary testing is the simplest way to examine cortisol's activity in its free, unbound form at the cellular level. Cortisol is a very potent hormone. Cortisol activity mediated by glucocorticoid receptors (GR), is tissue/organ specific and exquisitely regulated by the body, as we will see later.

I had a busy solo medical practice for many years. I recognized early on in my career that if I was going to work in a group practice, I would have to adhere to the allopathic values that guide western medicine. Flying solo is not a matter of temperament. It's fundamentally my protest against the narrow goals of a "medicine industrial complex" where insurance companies reimburse physicians for providing an approved set of services, but not necessarily for getting to the root cause of a patient's illness. Certainly, nobody was going to encourage me to throw myself into the study of cortisol!

Let me take a deeper dive here.

As a patient, you know the average office visit lasts about seventeen minutes. Seventeen minutes for your doctor to talk to you about your presenting complaints, assess your physical condition, and ask if anything else is bothering you. Within the same time span, your physician creates a treatment plan, discusses it with you, answers your questions, orders tests, prescribes medications, and populates your electronic health record (EHR). Under current healthcare reforms, medical competence has become a matter of checking off boxes in the EHR and complying with various metrics – some of which are not evidence-based – simply to satisfy the insurer's demands. A physician employed by a commercial medical group practice is all but forced into fetishizing productivity.

I knew I could be more effective if I went solo. And I have been. I do whatever is best for my patients. And if that takes me sixty or ninety minutes instead of seventeen, so be it. My approach to diagnosis does not stop at the symptom or illness level. I keep peeling away the layers of the onion to get to the problem at the cellular level.

My mindset is empathy. In our healthcare system, that's a non-billable commodity. I like talking to my patients. I like helping them get to the bottom of their physical and emotional needs.

Over time, as I began experiencing some of the conditions I s aw in my patients, my empathy with them grew even stronger. It was now clear to me that the source of my ailments lay in the same environmental problem that was afflicting my patients.

Stress!

Like so many doctors, I had succumbed to burnout. How was that possible? I love medicine, especially my chosen areas of specialization. How could *I* be overwhelmed?

I wasn't alone. Many of my physician colleagues and nurses were struggling with burnout too. They reported feeling emotionally exhausted. Their sense of personal achievement decreased. They were mortified to acknowledge negative attitudes toward the profession they once adored. Understanding that their burnout dovetailed with the ever-growing demands of regulatory compliance did not explain away their unhappiness.

Writing in the New England Journal of Medicine, Pamela Hartzband, MD, and Jerome Groopman, MD summed up physician burnout like this:

"The unintended consequences of radical alterations in the healthcare system that were supposed to make physicians more efficient and productive, and thus more satisfied, have made them profoundly alienated and disillusioned."[6]

Indeed, a 2022 survey of 13,000 physicians showed that about a fifth of those surveyed felt depressed. One in ten said they have thought about suicide or attempted it. Suicidal ideation was even more evident in female physicians, possibly because of their additional family responsibilities — and, I would add, because of their different response to stress.[7]

Evolutionarily speaking, the stress response is meant to protect us. Cortisol is an absolutely essential hormone — the savior in our "fight or flight" response to trouble. We can't live without it! Hans Selye, a pioneering endocrinologist who first described the HPA axis and general adaptation syndrome (to stress) in the 1940s, himself said, "Stress is the spice of life." So, let's not vilify cortisol! What matters is how we close the stress cycle.

Here's the paradox about cortisol. It can stay high for years and years. While excessive cortisol levels are not an expression of good health, a precipitate drop in cortisol can be even worse. Low cortisol levels lead to exhaustion and predispose you to a higher risk of mortality. Once your cortisol levels are severely low, they're much harder to fix. Not impossible — just harder. Sometimes physicians use the misleading terms "adrenal fatigue," or "adrenal exhaustion," to refer to low cortisol levels. Neither term actually reflects the body's complex mechanisms involved in adapting to chronic stress.[8] Since the adrenal glands are controlled by the brain via the Hypothalamic Pituitary Adrenal axis, a decreased cortisol output is most likely a down-regulation of the HPA axis to protect tissues from excess – and detrimental – cortisol. The correct terms used by clinicians and researchers are HPA axis dysfunction, hypocortisolism or hypercortisolism.

Our master hormone is a complicated, fascinating, and most misunderstood fellow!

In Western medicine, with its mission to alleviate the *symptoms* of disease through pharmaceuticals, you need to have either the extreme high (Cushing's), or the extreme low (Addison's), to be considered abnormal. In the personalized and functional medicine world, by contrast, your cortisol levels exist on a spectrum. What's measured as "normal" for one person may not be optimal for themselves, and may differ between people.

Let me be personal — because that is key to understanding what cortisol is doing in *your* body.

I have entered menopause, a known stressor on the body and mind of a woman. Like any chronic stressor, studies have shown that menopause raises the cortisol level.[9]

On top of menopause, I had a car accident. The resulting physical and emotional stress I dealt with only exacerbated the stress that comes along with a woman's "change of life." Add menopause and a car accident to the "ordinary" stresses of being a highly empathic doctor in solo medical practice, and the only child of elderly parents on the other side of the world? You have a perfect storm for burnout.

We'll get into the details of cortisol secretion a bit later, but suffice it to say for now that whenever our body secretes cortisol, DHEA and pregnenolone — two counter-regulatory hormones — are secreted too. As burnout-related stress becomes more chronic, the counter-regulatory hormones begin to fail. What happens next is not pretty: Cortisol starts to break down bone and muscle. To add insult to injury, it increases your body's visceral fat deposits.[10] And it shrinks the hippocampus, a part of the limbic system in the brain involved in learning, spatial processing, and memory. A healthy hippocampus is needed in feedback regulation of the HPA axis for dampening the stress response.[11]

As one-half of this book's writing team, I am one of the right people to write about cortisol. My patients come in with physiological and mental health problems directly related to the cortisol levels in their bodies. Those problems may present as resistance to weight loss, poor nighttime sleep, gastrointestinal issues, and/or depression, to name a few common symptoms. Guess what? I am intimately familiar with some of these symptoms as well.

As a gastroenterologist, I pay close attention to the health of the gut wall and the microbiome — the gut's trillions of microbes that break down toxins, synthesize vitamins, and defend against infection. Almost everything affects the health and well-being of the microbiome: Our food intake, our sleep habits, our daily exercise, our work, even our social status. All of these factors are shaped by stress! When my patients or I put on weight or when we feel excessively fatigued, I put cortisol under the microscope, so to speak. Because when you bathe your gut in cortisol, the bad bugs in there are going to have a party.

The cortisol-measuring technology Wibe and his team have created will give me a tool to help my patients and myself solve a medical puzzle. You see, so much of medical practice is — or should be — about solving our healthcare problems. Let's circle back to my reason for working in healthcare as a solo practitioner: I want to be part of the solution. I do not want to do harm. I reject putting my expertise, my intellect, and my healing abilities at the service of a broken medical system that processes people like factory widgets. I am grateful that, with my training and my mindset, I have helped people live more fulfilling and healthier lives because *I also check their cortisol levels.*

Wibe here.

Ioana, the pleasure is mine. Working on an immense problem – alongside a medical expert – is a thrill. It combines my love of technology and my commitment to improving life for millions of people.

Our brains haven't kept up with the algorithms – largely at the core of social media – that are managing our daily lives. Anxiety, depression, and stress are all up. Connecting, person to person in real life, is down. Our phones are our dinnertime companions! Paradoxically, Pardigm also uses a phone and algorithms to address a serious issue in our lives. Wasting time on your phone can create stress, but spending it wisely can help you control stress, weight, and many other physical and emotional problems.

Pardigm's app is not just a better technical way to measure cortisol. It also empowers you to take control of your own health and wellness. With a healthy cortisol rhythm, your body will be more resilient to stressors such as lost sleep and psychosocial pressures. It's up to us – the partnership between science and technology – to make the testing easier, affordable, and real-time. We'll give you the means to be proactive in your health that you haven't had until now.

Do we want chronically elevated cortisol to break down our defenses one at a time? Or do we want to take destiny into our own hands? As Ioana makes it clear, some forms of stress, managed well, can be a good thing.[12] Let's keep in mind that the evolutionary goal of the stress response is to help boost the body and mind into enhanced functioning. It exists to help us meet the environmental demands we face. But in a world where a work deadline or a failing relationship is a more likely stressor than a panther in your backyard grasslands, this non-specific stress response becomes maladaptive.

If I sound like a results-driven dreamer, I'm proud to say that's exactly what I aim to be. I don't do things by half-measures. I see the value in quantifying the mind-body connection. Our time in this world is short, and we want to eliminate cortisol imbalance as a leading cause of early death. [13] The reality is, high cortisol levels strongly predict cardiovascular death among people with *and without* preexisting cardiovascular disease, indicating that high cortisol levels are damaging to the cardiovascular system. The top drugs prescribed to adults in the US are mostly for diseases in which stress plays first or second violin. The result: serious problems with our immune system, insulin sensitivity, leaky gut, depression, sleep, sexual health, and blood pressure, to enumerate a few.[14]

And how about longevity? According to Dr. Elissa Epel at the University of California, San Francisco, "Cortisol reactivity has predicted telomere[15] shortening and both higher and lower cortisol have been linked with shorter telomeres.[16][17][18][19][20]? Telomere shortening is a key predictor of mortality and diseases among many other health issues.[21]

I'm adding attention deficit hyperactivity disorder (ADHD) to the list due to a recent study in *Nature*.[22] Would modern kids need to be on Adderall, Ritalin, and Prozac if they had healthy cortisol levels?

I spent my technology career in the mobile and artificial intelligence (AI) industries. I consider my years with Gillette, Nokia, and Huuuge a prerequisite course for solving the rapid test issue without the need for a lab. With a dozen PhDs in Computer Vision – an AI field that lets computers derive meaningful information from digital images and other visual inputs – we developed a phone app that can read your test results without the need for a lab scanner or any other device. Then we teamed up with the best scientists, doctors, and biochemists in the world to test the solution.

I have a lot of skin in the technology game. I'm putting that same skin in the biomarker technology game. Yet my passion for this project takes its inspiration from a family member under a psychiatrist's care. I asked the psychiatrist, "How do you quantify stress?"

Sadly, the reply was not reassuring: "We ask the patient how they feel."

Feelings are unquestionably important, but they should not be the only basis for quantifying physical or psychological disease.

I said, "That's not good enough."

I came to see that scientists have known for decades that cortisol is the gold standard biomarker for stress, energy, and recovery. Establishing a baseline for cortisol levels, which naturally vary in a specific pattern throughout the day, however, was the grand challenge. The time was right for me, personally, to apply my cross-industry expertise.

I went on a quest to quantify stress. I didn't know much about cortisol at first. I did know, though, that focusing almost exclusively on qualitative issues, such as "feelings," was not useful in a data-driven world. No pun intended: A qualitative approach to mental health, to the exclusion of quantitative evidence, is just insane.

Even the burnout Ioana talks about: Why don't we have a quantitative way of talking about it? I echo what Ioana says about cortisol in relation to our physical, emotional and cognitive health: *Doctors need to bring the qualitative in line with the quantitative.*

As somebody who sees emotional suffering in his own family, I want everybody to have the tools to be healthy and perform at their best.

The entrepreneur in me says: "Hey, there's a beautiful opportunity here to develop a product that already has a destination. All we need to do is to build the vehicle to get there."

GET TO KNOW US BECAUSE WE WANT TO KNOW YOU

We're going to build market awareness around cortisol.

If that sounds like a tall order, think about how undereducated people were about insulin, say, ten years ago. That's not the case anymore. Today we have continuous glucose monitors that do, in essence, what we want our cortisol home test to do: Give us a data-rich picture of cortisol's effect on infertility, menopausal symptoms, athletic recovery, burnout, weight loss resistance, cancer therapy response, longevity – and the list goes on.

Ioana talked about her love of solving puzzles. We're two peas in a pod.

The first business puzzle for me was, "Can we replace a hugely expensive lab scanner with an iPhone or Android that has a high-quality camera sensor?" The second was, "How much competition is out there?" We didn't want to build another mousetrap.

My team and I did six months of market, medical, and technological research before we said, "We're ready to build a startup."

Sounds easy? It wasn't!

I had to convince myself that of all the ideas or products I could invest in, resolving the cortisol issue was the most important project I could take on.

Still, why me and not somebody else?

First, a rookie entrepreneur would have a hard time building out a solution on the scale we're talking about. A newbie isn't necessarily equipped to upset a multi-billion-dollar healthcare industry that relies on expensive lab testing. Failing at a few startups, as I have done, really helps put things in perspective. So does my experience on a team that took another startup all the way to an IPO.

Second, a medical or biotech team usually does not have the experience to define the go-to-market strategy. Medical researchers are brilliant at what they do, but building a computer vision model takes a team of AI experts with a range of computing disciplines complemented by user experience, and marketing strategies. You need to know what the boundaries are — and then you need to know how to bust them. I can check the box on that one! I was the first to build a mobile artificial intelligence bot — a computer program that simulates a human activity — and the first to build an online video game on a mobile platform. AI bots are already aiding doctors in the diagnosis of many conditions. Why not leverage AI technology to test cortisol?

What my team is doing with our cortisol-measuring technology resembles what the Internet did to the retail industry: It *disintermediated* the need for brick-and-mortar stores. My team is *disintermediating* the need for a physical bio lab. Eliminating the middleman between producers and consumers will put healthcare directly in the hands of doctors and patients – with instant results. The benefits to healthcare consumers are enormous. The savings to the healthcare industry are all but incalculable.

We don't want to get ahead of ourselves, but once we have an inexpensive, simple-to-use, easily available cortisol-measuring technology, we're essentially building a platform that will work for measuring other hormones and biomarkers such as estrogen, testosterone, Vitamin D, uric acid, progesterone, and thyroid hormones. Ioana can vouch that progesterone and uric acid are detectable in saliva — every bit as much as cortisol is. Think what measuring progesterone, a hormone necessary for the implantation of a fertilized egg in the uterus, will do for women suffering from infertility issues. They can reach for their phone and measure it at home. Think how measuring uric acid, a marker for inflammation, metabolic health, and conditions leading to premature death, will help us make healthier dietary and lifestyle decisions.[23]

These other test formats can wait. Right now measuring cortisol holds the key to unlocking a massive number of healthcare problems. More than any other biomarker, it will make a profound difference in the health of the world's population.

Let's address the elephant in the room.

Theranos CEO Elizabeth Holmes became famous for making *unsubstantiated* claims that analyzing a single blood droplet would yield actionable information about dozens of medical conditions. Her purported analytical device, however, received Federal Drug Administration approval only for testing herpes. Even here the FDA noted that the device was "substantially equivalent" to existing technology, and for that reason no obstacle stood in the way of marketing it. Sorry, but you cannot market a sham product and expect it to upend a branch of medicine that provides data for some 70 percent of medical decisions.

Our team does not have to grandstand. To date, taking a picture of a test strip with our iPhone is becoming on par with lab scanners that most diagnostic labs in the world use. We expect our phone sensors to allow an even higher level of accuracy in the future.[24]

I'd like to share something a lot of people probably don't know about me.

I started a foundation to get underprivileged kids into college with the help of academic tutoring, sports training, and community service. I founded another foundation to save the last few endangered saolas in Laos and Vietnam.

This is my way of saying, "It's not all about the money."

It was inevitable that as I entered midlife — a time to reflect gratefully on the advantages and achievements that brought me to my present state — I would turn my attention to healthcare. I'm one of those GenXers driven to leave the planet a better place than I found it.

Ioana, our team, and I are pioneers in the use of affordable technology to tackle the world's biggest problems. We think that innovation, perseverance, and expertise are our only options.

Let's move on to see how measuring cortisol and other biomarkers will make life better for everyone in every corner of our planet – simply and in real time.

If you're going to dream, dream big.

Chapter 2

Why You Should Measure Your Cortisol Levels

As the Goldilocks principle[1] tells us, a good life is all about finding what fits just right. The same is true about our cortisol levels. Too high or too low is unhealthy. In fact, both conditions have been linked to a multitude of mental and physical ailments, including the shortening of the DNA's telomeres, the protective covering at the ends of our chromosomes. Diminished telomeres, whether from a genetic predisposition or stress, accelerate the aging process. For those of us who want to reach super-old age, that's terrifying to hear. If you knew your cortisol levels were out of balance – and threatened to age you faster than normal – wouldn't you want to take steps to get them "just right?"

Living long and well is the best reason to measure your cortisol levels. As "levels" indicates, one number alone isn't sufficient to understand the impact of cortisol on your body. Because cortisol levels fluctuate throughout the day, you and your doctor need to see the hormone's numbers mapped over a 24-hour circadian, naturally recurring, cycle.

The Cortisol Awakening Response (CAR), for example, measures the cortisol level change between the moment you open your eyes to the light and 30 minutes post-wake-up. A high CAR is associated with stress and negative anticipation for upcoming events. A low CAR is associated with PTSD, burnout, and systemic dysregulation – all chronic conditions.[2] Both of these "not just right" levels are associated with poor health outcomes.

Let's take a look at normal cortisol diurnal rhythm measurements, as well as several unhealthy patterns you'd want to address.[3,4]

CORTISOL: THE MASTER HORMONE

CAR = cortisol awakening response. Cortisol is measured in saliva in ng/mL.

Categories	CAR	Afternoon	Evening
Cortisol in balance	OK	OK	OK
Cortisol chronically elevated	High	High	High
Cortisol high CAR	High	OK	OK
Cortisol elevated dropping in the evening	High	High	OK
Cortisol small afternoon peak	OK	High	OK
Cortisol small evening peak	OK	OK	High
Cortisol low throughout	Low	Low	Low
Cortisol midday steep drop	OK	Low	OK

LET'S TAKE A GRANULAR LOOK AT EACH CATEGORY.

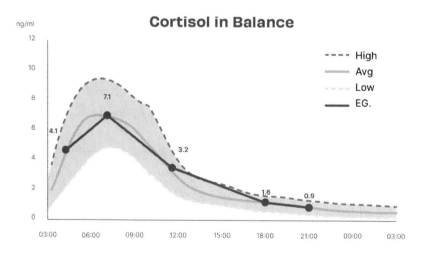

When you're healthy, your cortisol spikes rapidly upon awakening, leading to a maximum peak (50-150% rise) about 30 minutes after waking up. This morning rise, called Cortisol Awakening Response or CAR, reflects the circadian rhythm of cortisol secre-

WHY YOU SHOULD MEASURE YOUR CORTISOL LEVELS

tion and is not induced, but can be affected, by stress. Cortisol then comes down throughout the day, more rapidly within the first 2-3 morning hours, and is the lowest at bedtime, allowing for smaller spikes when you're stressed. The low value in the evening gets you ready for bed, and is required for melatonin[5] secretion. The high spike in the morning wakes you up and prepares you for the day.

This optimal cortisol rhythm – visible in the green range – exists when there's no interference from perceived stress, trauma, poor sleep, unhealthy BMI, or drugs affecting the HPA axis. Exercise or a heavy meal with a high glycemic index will cause a cortisol spike, but, in a healthy person, the balance is restored within ~ two hours. The CAR/morning reading serves as a "stress test of the coming (anticipatory) or previous day."

Cortisol pattern: elevated throughout the day

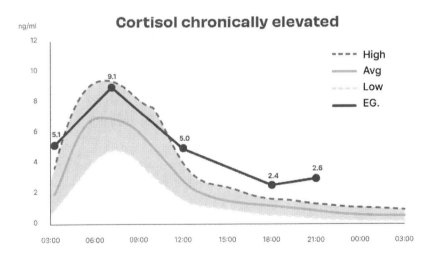

Even a 10% or 20% increase in cortisol levels throughout the day will have a major impact on your body and mind. When you're stressed, it's common to crave sugar and other carbs, feel "tired but wired," have trouble sleeping, and/or feel anxiety. This can lead to other hormone imbalances. Progesterone will be suppressed down? and women can experience spotting, abdominal pain, and fatigue. Men will have suppressed testosterone and can experience erectile dysfunction, and fatigue.

A "flat line" elevated level with no diurnal variation is suggestive of Cushing's disease and should be investigated by your physician.

What we recommend

Elsewhere we'll discuss how to refocus your mindset so you can improve your coping skills – and thereby decrease your stress.

Keep your blood sugar stable. Limit your daily coffee intake and alcohol.

Don't overdo your exercise, and expect a cortisol spike after intense training, done preferably in the morning.

Make sure you go to bed early. No electronic distractions![6]

Cortisol pattern: high early morning/ or elevated CAR only

When your cortisol level in the morning is above the normal range, it's usually a sign of perceived/anticipatory job stress that can be more pronounced during week-day and closer to normal during the week-ends. A muscle ache, a tough workout, or a poor night's sleep will register in the morning as elevated cortisol. It's also the first step toward depression.[7] Be aware that cortisol levels increase with age.

WHY YOU SHOULD MEASURE YOUR CORTISOL LEVELS

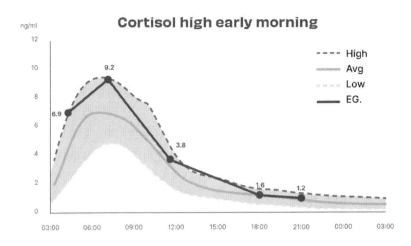

What we recommend

Focus on your sleep by implementing rigorous bedtime rituals. These will help ensure sufficient, high-quality sleep.

During the week, schedule time for activities you enjoy (hobbies, reading, movies, pets, friends). All work and no play creates the conditions for depression.

Try to focus your exercise in the morning, on strength-training and cardio.[8] In the US, cardiometabolic health has been declining: Only 6.8% of adults have optimal cardiometabolic health. Stress can result in adverse effects on the body composition, even in young, apparently healthy individuals, because cortisol and the autonomic nervous system control the three body composition compartments – muscle, fat and bone.

Cortisol pattern: elevated cortisol with evening drop

With prolonged stress, your cortisol levels will be higher than normal throughout the day. Stressful events are the cause. Sometimes food consumption and exercise are too. It's likely you'll crave sugar, carbs, salt, fat and other "comfort" food.

Your sleep will be impacted and you might feel anxious.

Progesterone is used to make cortisol, so progesterone levels drop when the body is under stress for extended periods – while cortisol levels rise.

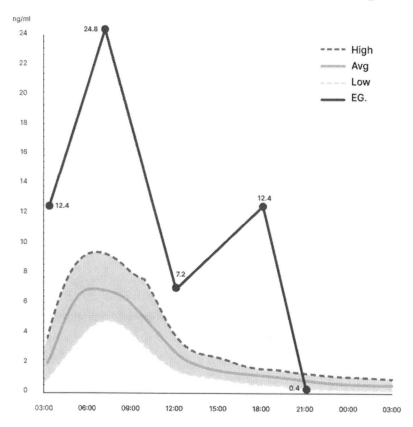

What we recommend

Eat protein three times a day: Protein supplies the body with amino acids to head off stress-induced cravings. Sorry, no snacking in between meals. Drink plenty of water and tea. Skip soft drinks and limit your coffee intake.

Do your work-outs in the morning – ideally 30 minutes of aerobic exercise along with some strength-training. Train yourself to go to bed early enough to accommodate your workout.

Read Chapter 10 on mindsets. Your goal is to reorient your thinking from a "stress is harmful" mindset to a "stress is enhancing" mindset. You'll find that the switch will help improve your coping skills.

Cortisol pattern: afternoon rebound

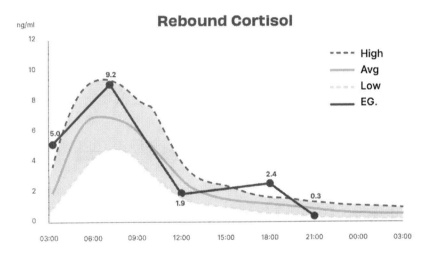

A small peak later in the day – not related to food or intense exercise – suggests that your energy levels vary throughout the day. You may experience symptoms in the morning or evening, such as fatigue, anxiety, irritability, poor concentration, impatience, and cravings.

"Afternoon rebound cortisol pattern" is different from a similar effect after exercise.[9] After exhaustive endurance exercise, however, cortisol could remain depressed for 24 - 48 hours.[10]

What we recommend

Try to exercise in the morning.

Hydrate well with enough water and tea. Cut down on carbs and caffeine. No soft drinks. If you don't get seven or eight hours of sleep, make sure you catch up over the next few days.

Cortisol pattern: elevated in evening

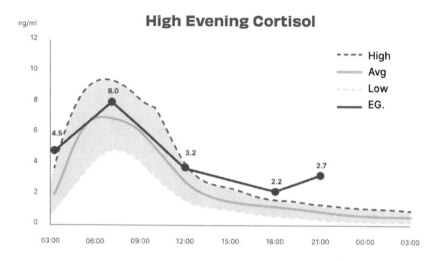

Higher levels in the evening and night indicate problems with your circadian rhythm. You might have trouble falling asleep, or you might be waking up in the middle of the night. Your body will feel pulled in two directions at the same time: Drained of energy but overly stimulated. Others might notice overly apprehensive or irritable behavior.

What we recommend

If your cortisol levels are still high at bedtime, curtail your exercise in the late afternoon or early evening. Cut down on

WHY YOU SHOULD MEASURE YOUR CORTISOL LEVELS

coffee early and move to tea and water throughout the day. Avoid alcohol, especially in the evening.

Set regular bedtime and wake-up times (and stick to them). Lower your bedroom temperature. Avoid electronics during the hours before bedtime (see footnote #2).

See supplementation recommendations in Chapter 11.

Cortisol pattern: low throughout the day

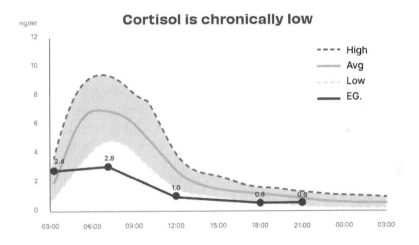

Low cortisol levels throughout the day indicate exhaustion, acute severe stress or recurrent infection. As we'll show later in the book, Long Covid is associated with chronically low cortisol, or hypocortisolism.

You wake up with no energy, have brain fog, dizziness, poor appetite and poor mood. Most likely you don't sleep without interruption. The rest of the day is also flattened, which might have an impact on your allergies and immune system.

A flattened diurnal curve with loss of CAR should be investigated with your doctor to rule out Addison's.

What we recommend

This is the most difficult pattern to fix. It usually requires supplementation and you might need guidance from a knowledgeable health practitioner.

Work on your mindset by embracing your stress (see Chapter 10). You're stressed about something you care about. Reconnect with the thing you care about.

Make sure your bedroom is completely dark. If ambient light is coming through your windows, invest in some blackout blinds. They're incredibly effective. Lower the room's temperature.[11] Take little naps during the day.

Go outside or expose yourself to natural light devices soon after you wake up to re-establish your circadian rhythm.

Cut the sugar and refined carbs in your diet and normalize blood sugar. Eat a complete, nutritious diet and don't skip meals (yet).

Do light restorative exercise in the morning, but don't overdo it.

Elite athletes should consider taking a few weeks off to let the body *and* mind recover.

Cortisol pattern: midday steep drop

A midday drop is normal, but if the drop is bigger than usual, it might indicate fatigue.

If you're exercising in the morning, you want your cortisol to drop – but not too much because you need to keep your glucose levels stable. If glucose isn't stable, your energy level will drop off. If the drop is severe, you'll crave sugar and caffeine.

WHY YOU SHOULD MEASURE YOUR CORTISOL LEVELS

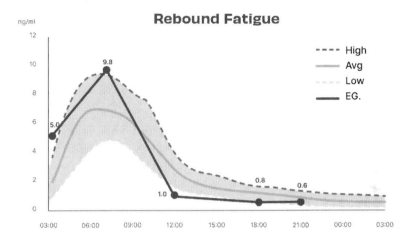

What we recommend

You'll want to reduce stress and improve your coping skills (see Chapter 10 on mindsets). Reduce the amount of refined carbs to keep your blood sugar stable. Definitely have protein at each meal. Don't skip lunch. Eat a nutritious diet.

Reduce caffeine. Drink plenty of water throughout the day. Herbal teas are great. Avoid soft drinks.

Get at least 7 hours of sleep and take catnaps. Get a boost by exercising mid-morning with a combination of muscle-building and cardiovascular activities. Schedule time for pleasurable activities.

Just by looking at cortisol's abnormal patterns, you can see we measure cortisol levels for one main reason: We want to manage results. Why do we want to do that? We want to take action to restore ourselves to good health, or what the body experiences as homeostasis — a constantly self-adjusting process by which our internal systems maintain the stability we need to survive.

How important is cortisol?

"If you take away the body's capacity to synthesize cortisol, either by removing the adrenal gland, the hypothalamus, or the pituitary gland, you would probably die within one day," says Netherlands-based endocrinologist Sjoerd van den Berg. "It is that important."

Cortisol is produced from cholesterol through multiple enzymatic steps by specialized cells in the outer portion of the adrenal glands, small triangular-shaped structures situated on top of the kidneys. It's secreted for at least two reasons: As a basal level it controls numerous homeostatic maintenance functions and keeps the body aligned with our circadian clock – a natural process that regulates our sleep–wake cycle and repeats roughly every 24 hours. And it serves as a stress response at critical moments when our body perceives the need to respond to danger.

The stress, via the HPA axis, induces cortisol secretion at critical moments when your body needs to respond to danger in order to : (1) increase in energy availability via glucose metabolism; (2) control blood pressure; (3) reduce inflammation and (4) increase alertness and memory encoding of the stressful experience.

To this end, it's crucial that we learn (1) the reason for our elevated or low cortisol, and (2) what constitutes normal cortisol levels and rhythm for each one of us.

Your doctor or nurse may already have measured your cortisol, usually by looking at your blood. Going this route to determine cortisol concentrations in the blood is not problem-free. First, collecting a blood sample is stressful and the procedure itself can up your cortisol level. Second, a blood test is typically done once a day, in the morning with the patient fasting. The blood draw will tell you the cortisol level at that moment only, but not at noon, or 3:00 p.m., or after dinner. Third, and critically important, most cortisol (90% or more) in the blood is bound to proteins – mainly corticosteroid-binding globulin (CBG) and, to a lesser extent, albumin. These proteins shuttle cortisol in a bound, inactive form around the body. When CBG and albumin levels are abnormal, as can happen in pregnancy, or liver and kidney diseases, they compromise the accurate measurement of cortisol. What we are most interested in is the free, unbound, biologically active fraction of cortisol that acts in body tissues.

Between one and ten percent of unbound cortisol can be measured in the blood, but it is too labor-intensive for routine clinical use. Blood measurements don't give us sufficiently detailed and reliable results.[12,13,14,15] According to Thomas Guilliams, Ph.D., "The calculated measure of free serum cortisol has been mostly replaced by salivary cortisol in both research and clinical practice, a measurement which effectively mirrors the serum-free fraction of cortisol."[16]

What about urinalysis? It has three distinct advantages over blood sampling: First, cortisol not bound to proteins — the cortisol we need to test — is "bioavailable" in your urine. Second, urinalysis depends on samples taken every time you pee, a plus when it comes to evaluating cortisol levels throughout the day. Third, urine is relatively easy to collect. You don't need any advanced training to do it.

Yet, there's a significant drawback to urinalysis stemming from the quality of the urine at time of collection, and what it measures: Urinary cortisol output reflects an average of the time, usually a few hours, since the previous urine void. Hence, morning urine reflects overnight cortisol production. Your next collection would tell you the level of cortisol in your urine since awakening. This collection, of course, may also be several hours out of date and would not provide the CAR data. In short, that first urine collection will likely show cortisol levels that are lower than the second one. But what are your cortisol levels right this minute when the mood you're in, or the food you've eaten, or the anxiety you feel at school or the office, has actually driven your cortisol levels up?

Cortisol in the saliva reflects the amount of free, bioactive cortisol (not bound to proteins). Optimally speaking, this cortisol, which enters tissues throughout the body and binds to cortisol receptors (GR= glucocorticoid and MR=mineralocorticoid receptors) to do the work, is the cortisol we want to measure. Free cortisol enters the saliva by diffusion, and quickly and reliably parallels changes in plasma cortisol concentration. Collecting your saliva five times throughout the day gives you and your expert consultant a picture of cortisol's longitudinal behavior in your body. This picture, which we saw above, is called the diurnal cortisol curve. Most salivary tests rely on four measurements during the day to create the diurnal cortisol curve. We recommend five measurements on Day 1 for everyone to also include the CAR. Depending on the case - for athletes, women suffering from infertility or women entering perimenopause with severe symptoms - we want even more data points over an extended period of time – a few months, for example. One baseline picture may not give us enough information, because cortisol is such a complex and changing actor.

All three of these cortisol testing options will give you an idea of cortisol's impact on your body and mind. Only the saliva test, however, will give you the quickest and most reliable reading. It also happens to be the easiest mode of testing available to date.[17]

"If a salivary test performs well, you'll reduce the costs associated with laboratory testing," says van den Berg. "You spare the patient a trip to the hospital or phlebotomy clinic. But most important, multiple testing on multiple days, by the patient, would make a smartphone testing device a sufficiently reliable source of accurate and precise data."

Van den Berg is not prepared to say that a phone app will absolutely replace lab testing. "The advantage of home salivary testing is that now you have a way to find disease fast and early," he says.

WHY YOU SHOULD MEASURE YOUR CORTISOL LEVELS

Now we know what type of cortisol test you should get. But why look at your cortisol levels at all?

If you're feeling bummed out, or you're experiencing low energy, or you're having trouble getting pregnant, or you're gaining too much weight, or your blood sugar levels are going through the roof — or you're having any number of other physiological or emotional problems — checking your cortisol levels will help you and your doctor figure out what's going wrong. Then you can figure out your next step. Succinctly put, the inciting factor is stress — the "health epidemic of the twenty-first century," according to the World Health Organization (2017). Our remote ancestors had to deal with the stress of a potential wild animal attack, or a drought-induced famine, or the premature death of a protector, and nobody would want to diminish the terror associated with these conditions. Yet, the stress we experience in our current technologically advanced world comes at us from every direction: Our Family life. The workplace. Our commute. Our search for a mate. The loss of a loved one. Financial pressures. Sociologists would add social stressors such as war, racism, ethnic hatred, food deserts, gun violence, and relentless political divisiveness. Epidemiologists would include the COVID-19 pandemic, which single-handedly wreaked havoc on people's finances and personal relationships for at least two years.

Stunningly, some 60-to-80 percent of all primary care doctor visits have a stress-related component. And the top ten drugs prescribed in the First World typically treat high blood pressure, high cholesterol, inflammation, thyroid malfunction, stomach acid, insomnia, and diabetes, to name only a few diseases linked directly to stress and high cortisol levels. Do not expect conventional physicians to check cortisol patterns, most frequently they don't know that a single measurement doesn't mean anything.

Let's be fair: We're grateful for access to pharmaceutical treatments. We don't want to underestimate their role in prolonging life and healing the body. But all too often, they arrive after disease has set in. That's too late. Treating disease symptoms is like putting a coat of paint on a structurally compromised house. For a less drug-dependent, more holistic approach to health, we want to address root problems.

Measuring your cortisol levels is a way to do that. You'll locate the source of your stress. Once you know what stress is doing to virtually every aspect of your life, you and your doctor can talk about next steps. You'll have the emotional and intellectual wherewithal to get healthy. Maybe for the first time in your life.

We don't want to freak you out. That's not why we're listing all the things that can go wrong when cortisol runs amok. We do feel a responsibility though to be your wakeup call. Elevated cortisol levels will threaten your quality of life and your longevity. They'll contribute to "brain melt," or cognitive deficiencies. They'll throw your metabolism out of whack. They'll interfere with your sex drive and your ability to produce sex hormones. They'll hobble your athletic prowess. They'll suppress your immune system. They'll atrophy your muscles and your bones.

No doubt you see people in your own life who have been beaten down by one infirmity or another. We're convinced cortisol has played a starring role in their deterioration. It doesn't have to be that way. And it won't be if you understand that cortisol runs the show. You've just got to get the shepherd's hook and pull that bad actor off the stage – and into its rightful place.

Step 1: Measure!

One more factor plays a role in the measurement and management of your cortisol levels, and that's affordable digital technology. Blood and urine tests typically depend on high-priced laboratory analysis for results. Salivary testing of the sort we advocate requires a test strip, a smartphone and an app.

Poor healthcare industry! It's mostly been a laggard when it comes to changing its processes and machinery to keep up with the times. Maybe that's as it should be. Good physicians are thoughtful. They deliberate over options. We remember as far back as the mid-1990s when medical offices were just starting to move from paper to electronic medical records. Doctors and nurses were reluctant to give up the tried and true, and they worried that learning computer programs would take time away from their core purpose. For most, it did. "Healthcare Information Technology-related stress is measurable, common (about 70% among practicing physicians respondents), specialty-related, and independently predictive of burnout symptoms".[18] But fast-forward a quarter of a century — and most ten-year-olds are computer-savvy. That's largely because of intuitive digital technologies, which have put everything from banking to gaming at the service of your thumbs.

Technology is not an obstacle anymore. When well designed, it's your companion. That's why every high-profile industry out there is defined by its app.

Retail. Banking. Ride-hailing. Food delivery. Fitness. Entertainment, film, news, and podcasting. Communications and social media. Education, books, and libraries. Financial investment. Weather forecasting. Payment systems. Maps. Parking.

We're adding rapid healthcare testing and results to the digital mix.

Ease-of-use alone is not enough, and we understand what's at stake if you get digital healthcare wrong. In fact, one word might sum up the anxiety the healthcare industry suffers when it comes to putting its eggs in the digital tech basket.

Theranos.

"I've been in the diagnostics industry long enough to truly understand how hard it is," says Tyler Schultz, a biotech researcher, entrepreneur, and whistleblower in the Theranos scandal. "The technological hurdles are high, the regulatory landscape is challenging, and the customer acquisition cost is profound. In short, you need rock-solid technology and a big, accessible market."

We'll argue that any biomarker company should also reject hype as a business strategy. The mindset we embrace involves scientific integrity and a good dose of humility. Every entrepreneur seeking to develop a disruptive technology experiences missteps, misdirections, glitches, failures. But when you have a development team committed to scrutinizing data and processes —a team that adheres to the scientific method — you're on a careful path to building a safe, ethical product. The ability to recognize a flaw is not admitting defeat. It underscores the rigor you bring to your project.

Indeed, the work is hard and the obstacles are not insignificant. That's why we respect guidelines established by the Federal Drug Administration (FDA), which assert that by measuring biomarkers in the body, biomarker technology promises to "reduce stagnation and foster innovation in the development of new medical products." We concur with the US federal agency when it observes that the "success of personalized medicine fundamentally depends on the development of biomarkers and diagnostic tests that can be used to accurately identify the patient population."[19]

Shultz says, "Having a tool to test for a biomarker, such as cortisol, in real-time lets you put together pieces of a biological puzzle."

Other researchers in the field of biological stress agree. "New technologies might get developed that will make cortisol home tests as widespread as COVID tests were in 2021," says Liesbeth Van Rossum, professor of medicine at Erasmus University Medical Center and renowned researcher on obesity and stress.[20]

What's important is the momentum a cortisol-measuring app can bring about in the biomarker measuring field: Pardigm and comparable development teams can lead the way to other biomarker measuring tools for uric acid, testosterone, estrogen, progesterone, and thyroid hormones, to name a few. The difference: these tests can produce quantitative results in real time.[21]

We'll get there. Methodically. Responsibly. Bad science and sloppy technology only temporarily create a black hole in the digital healthcare marketplace. Good science and ever-sophisticated technology remind us that biomarker diagnostics are within our reach when we work with talented, analytical teams to answer these questions: What's the problem? What biomarker should we test? Based on test results, what's the optimal treatment? What's the right therapy for this particular person?

Therein lies the true value of measuring your cortisol.

TAKEAWAYS

- Cortisol is the Master Hormone: it is essential to life, and the body will prioritize making cortisol over all other hormones.

- Hormones are essential messengers in your body that tell your cells what to do and when to do it. They work in concert, so you cannot have an isolated hormonal imbalance. Cortisol has the strongest voice in influencing other hormones.

- You cannot achieve true health without balancing your cortisol. Abnormal cortisol patterns profoundly affect almost every process in your body, from your energy production and metabolism, immune function, brain and mental health, to your weight, digestion and reproduction.

- Out-of-balance cortisol is reversible -- and you can take the right steps to reverse it when you measure it. Correcting your cortisol rhythm is much easier than living with the effects of abnormal cortisol patterns.

- The easiest and most effective way to measure your cortisol levels is with home-based salivary tests, however, there are no real-time tests on the market today. Pardigm[22] is filling that void by placing the power to measure and manage cortisol in your hands.

Chapter 3

How Monitoring Cortisol Can Help Manage Burnout, Stress and Mental Disorders

You won't find "burnout" in the Diagnostic and Statistical Manual of Mental Disorders V (DSM V), a rather unsatisfactory labeling catalog of psychiatric conditions that health professionals use to characterize mental disorders. Burnout is consigned to a somewhat diffuse category of "undifferentiated somatoform disorder." That's because the current state of science suggests that burnout is a form of depression, not an illness in its own right. Wherever burnout belongs in the psychiatric register, the phenomenon is widespread and serious: It's been associated with a loss of $322 billion a year in job turnover and lower productivity.[1] The people said to suffer the most from it are often the best and the brightest in the global workplace. They're among the most dedicated workers who put in long hours in a quest to "give back" to society. When their best-laid plans go off the rails, they blame themselves. They're like the frog in slowly boiling water: By the time they've given their all, they're already "boiling over" with emotional exhaustion, cynicism, and self-blame.

Workplace fatigue, as a psychological and physiological concept, caught fire in the early 1970s, when psychoanalyst Herbert Freudenberger coined the term "burnout syndrome." In *Burnout: The High Cost of High Achievement*, which Freudenberger published in 1974, he observed that individuals, committed heart and soul to a cause or relationship, lose motivation when their actions fail to produce the desired results. Freudenberger based his insights on himself and his colleagues working with chronic drug abusers and other clinical populations. Along with social psychologists, Christina Maslach and Susan E. Jackson, who designed the Maslach Burnout Inventory Scale, Freudenberger came to see that love of work and dedication to a cause didn't protect mental health professionals from experiencing low morale, skipping out on work, and even providing subpar quality of care. Indeed, Freudenberger's own fifteen-hour work days, spent working in the free drug treatment clinics he set up in San Francisco, left him and his colleagues intimately acquainted with the symptoms of burnout: cardiovascular disease, musculoskeletal pain, depression, job dissatisfaction, and absenteeism, to name a few.[2]

Burnout can affect anybody in any workplace, but the ideal candidate is a people person. The typical candidate for burnout is a healthcare, social work, or human services professional — an individual who spends considerable time in face-to-face contact with people who need help. Often this sort of interaction focuses on the client's immediate problem, which is psychological, social, physical, or financial, and is typically fraught with a range of intense emotions. For people who work day-in-day-out with such clients, chronic stress is an ever-present reality. The demands of the job can become so severe that the therapists, doctors, and others who went into their profession to help people now find themselves confronting feelings of callousness, depersonalization, even anger toward clients. They may even succumb to an alternate phenomenon called "vicarious traumatization,"[3] where healthcare professionals who have worked with torture survivors, are prone to developing symptoms of post-traumatic stress disorder, or manifest "compassion fatigue."[4]

Like depression, burnout doesn't happen overnight. It builds up after repeated interactions with difficult personalities or situations, until it deserves to be called chronic stress. Freudenberger and North described 12 steps which lead to burnout, not always necessarily in the same order: the compulsion to prove oneself, working harder, dismissal of conflict, neglecting own needs, distortion of values, heightened denial, disengagement, observable behavioral changes, depersonalization, emptiness, depression and total burnout exhaustion. As we've seen with so many other manifestations of stress, burnout, too, registers as a perturbation of cortisol levels.

A Medical University of Vienna study of stress-specific biomarkers, for example, observed that at baseline, significantly higher levels of salivary cortisol were discovered in the burnout group compared to the control group of healthy individuals.[5] The research goal was not only to associate cortisol levels with burnout, but also to help burnout victims identify times of peak stress. Interestingly, researchers found that midday and end-of-day salivary cortisol readings especially aided in the assessment and bio-monitoring of burnout.

Let's review the physiological origin of the stress response. In the general population and in burnout sufferers, it's thought to begin in the brain's amygdala, an area that perceives the distress signal and relays it to the hippocampus, the brain's command center. From there, two events occur: a rapid response, via the sympathetic-adreno-medullar (SAM) axis, which releases epinephrine and norepinephrine within seconds; and a slow response, via the hypothalamus-pituitary-adrenal (HPA) axis, which results in the release of corticotropin-releasing hormone (CRH), a peptide hormone, from the hypothalamus. CRH, in turn, directs the pituitary gland to release adrenocorticotropic hormone (ACTH). The end result of this HPA axis activation is cortisol – produced by the adrenal cortex under the stimulating effect of ACTH. It peaks in the bloodstream, ready to save the day, 15-20 minutes after the initial stressor.

In short, hormonal signaling across the HPA axis wih increased CRH levels results in elevated cortisol in healthy individuals, and a maladaptive behavior with a blunted response, especially in the morning, in individuals with chronic depression or burnout.[6]

Back to the relationship between burnout and cortisol.

The Medical University of Vienna study of stress-specific biomarkers observed that at baseline, significantly higher levels of salivary cortisol were discovered in the burnout group from a preventive care ward — compared to the control group of healthy individuals. The research goal was not only to associate cortisol levels with burnout, but also to help burnout victims identify times of peak stress. Interestingly, researchers found that midday and end-of-day salivary cortisol readings especially aided in the assessment and bio-monitoring of burnout. (To a lesser extent, morning cortisol concentrations were useful biomarkers too.) Blood-borne biomarkers (IL-6, homocysteine and myeloperoxidase in this study) did not offer any significant predictive value. The multipronged treatment program resulted in a significant reduction of stress, anxiety, and depression scores with 60% of patients showing a clinically relevant improvement. This was accompanied by a ~30% drop in midday cortisol levels , as well as a ~25% decrease in end-of-day cortisol.

Just to complicate matters — and matters are always complicated where cortisol is concerned! — older adults in the Medical University of Vienna study, who suffered from depression (but not necessarily burnout), were found to display significantly higher levels of basal cortisol than the healthy control group during all cortisol testing phases throughout the day, and particularly during evening and night-time hours. Indeed, we know that cortisol levels in both men and women increase by 20-50% between the ages of 20 and 80. [7] And rumination — a mode of fixation that focuses on negative thoughts, past and present, and results in emotional distress — was shown to delay the cortisol decline during the day. Ruminative thinking and elevated cortisol levels in burnout victims may even contribute to sleep problems, which in turn, perturb cortisol levels throughout the day.[8]

Typically, however, low cortisol levels are associated with anxiety, PTSD, and burnout in people who have survived all kinds of super-high-stress situations. Low cortisol levels have also been found in the children of people who experienced trauma and chronic depression. In her evaluation of 187 pregnant women who had been in the area of the World Trade Center on September 11, 2001, for example, psychiatrist Rachel Yehuda and her team at Mount Sinai's Icahn School of Medicine in New York found that some of the women had developed post-traumatic stress disorder (PTSD) — as well as low levels of cortisol. "Surprisingly and disturbingly," she wrote in an essay describing how parental trauma leaves biological traces in children, "the saliva of the nine-month-old babies of women with PTSD also showed low cortisol. The effect was most prominent in babies whose mothers had been in their third trimester on that fateful day."

Yehuda was all the more astonished by her team's evaluation of the 9/11 pregnant women, which came only a year after the team she led reported low cortisol levels in adult children of Holocaust survivors. "We'd assumed that [the low cortisol levels] had something to do with being raised by parents who were suffering from the long-term emotional consequences of severe trauma," she wrote. "Now it looks like trauma leaves a trace in offspring even before they are born."

Yehuda's findings dovetailed with her work in the 1980s with a group of US military veterans. Indeed, she learned that ongoing stress associated with PTSD, as well as lower than normal cortisol levels, also appeared in US veterans of the Vietnam War.

"There was no question about it," Yehuda wrote. "Even if the traumatic experience was long ago, PTSD went hand in hand with low cortisol."

As Rachel Yehuda's longitudinal studies suggest, researchers have pondered the complicated relationship between cortisol and depression since the 1970s. What further complicates the research is the heterogeneous nature of depression. Indeed, Mario Juruena, MD, a researcher and clinical senior lecturer in translational psychiatry at King's College London, co-authored a review paper that compiled all the key research on the role cortisol plays in various kinds of depressive disorders. Because depression manifests as subtypes, and appropriate criteria defining these subtypes are still a matter of debate, the clinician or researcher's job is to analyze what kind of depression the patient exhibits. Dr. Juruena concluded unequivocally that the "link between abnormalities of the hypothalamic-pituitary-adrenal (HPA) axis and depression has been one of the most consistently reported findings in psychiatry."[9]

To gain an even deeper appreciation for the uniqueness of each depressive subtype, Dr. Juruena and his team reviewed all the research papers found in four scientific databases between 1946 and 2007. He found that the majority of studies confirmed the association between melancholic depression and increased cortisol levels – but the association with increases in basal cortisol and basal ACTH were less consistent. Juruena wrote that "our findings indicate that there is a difference in the HPA axis between melancholic and atypical depressive subtypes." Melancholia was associated with hypercortisolism (elevated cortisol levels) and atypical depression was associated with somewhat more normal cortisol levels .

Juruena and his colleagues plan on researching the relationship between cortisol and serotonin – the "feel-good" chemical that carries messages between brain nerve cells and the rest of the body and helps decrease anxiety.

"I really believe that the HPA axis is the control center for all the other neurotransmitter systems, not only the serotonergic system," Juruena says. "You know, if you are using benzodiazepines – a class of psychoactive drugs used to lower brain activity and to treat conditions such as anxiety, insomnia, and seizures – you are interfering with the HPA axis. The question is, what is the impact on the body when we do this? If you are above or below the optimal level of cortisol, you will be vulnerable to various kinds of mental or physical disorders, everything from asthma and diabetes to decreased libido."

Salivary cortisol

― Placebo - depression
- - Placebo - controls
― Prednisolone - depression
- - - Prednisolone - controls

09:00 12:00 17:00

Dr. Juruena holds out hope for ketamine and glucocorticoid receptor modulators to target treatment-resistant depression.

"It's amazing to see patients, who did not respond well to therapy or electroconvulsive therapy, respond favorably to ketamine, which works through the glutamatergic pathway," Juruena says. "I believe 50% - 60% of patients will benefit. Ketamine and drugs like it could be the next wave in treatment for HPA axis-related depression."

Cortisol, as the end-product of HPA axis reactivity, has an enormous influence on severe treatment-resistant depression. This graph, taken from one of Dr. Mario Juruena's seminal papers, shows elevated cortisol for groups with refractory depression – depression that does not respond to at least two medications. Here Dr. Juruena designed an improved HPA axis suppression test using prednisolone (a synthetic corticosteroid that binds to both glucocorticoid and mineralocorticoid receptors) to evaluate the HPA axis responsiveness in patients with psychiatric disorders.[10]

In studying trauma and cortisol levels, researchers are confronted with several questions about the relationship between cortisol and depression subtypes:

How is the chain of events leading up to burnout or any other depressive condition influenced by cortisol? Is there a way of knowing beyond a shadow of a doubt which comes first? The depressive symptoms or the change in cortisol? Moreover, once you experience burnout, can you recover from it? Can you prevent it in the first place?

Clearly, burnout has a sociological as well as a psychological profile, and Australian sociologist Celia Roberts and British medical sociologist Brigit McWade have advocated for a "sociology of stress" that would "take seriously the biological and physiological processes" inherent in disease. Such a discipline would involve a multifactorial approach to stress that goes beyond mere measurement, noting the complicating factor that "cortisol patterns may also refer to historic rather than present life circumstances."

While burnout is every bit as serious a condition as major

depressive disorder, PTSD, or any other mental health condition, people who suffer from burnout may have an advantage: With coaching, candidates for burnout can be on the alert for signs of workplace exhaustion, vicarious traumatization, and compassion fatigue.

Early Stress Life (ELS) - all traumatic experiences occurring before the age of 18, or a woman's first menstrual cycle,[11] - is also associated with abnormalities of the HPA axis. The impact of "early adversity" on the HPA axis's response to stress makes people vulnerable to both physical and psychiatric diseases in later life .[12]

Neuroendocrinologist Robert Sapolsky, described the nuanced effects of cortisol in the body,[13] and brilliantly explained in his book, " Why Zebras Don't Get Ulcers," mechanisms of stress response. Sapolsky reassures us that we can change the way we cope with stress, in the workplace and in our personal lives, physiologically and psychologically. Preparing to deal with workplace burnout and any other type of stress, however, isn't simply a matter of looking into a mirror and telling yourself, "I'm good enough, I'm smart enough, and doggone it, people like me!"[14] Sapolsky makes some straightforward recommendations:

Exercise. When you face burnout due to fraught workplace interactions, take time to exercise. A regular exercise regimen decreases your risk of various metabolic and cardiovascular diseases.

Meditate. If practiced on a regular basis, meditation decreases glucocorticoid levels. (At least one caveat: Studies show the physiological benefits while a person meditates. The good results, such as lowered blood pressure, may not endure very long.)

Find social support. The trick is to get social support from the right person, the right network of friends, the right community. If possible, be the one to give social support. That makes you feel needed and — in the best-case scenario — reduces your own feelings of stress-related social isolation.

Be humble. Find the wisdom to pick your battles. It's not a bad idea to contemplate Reinhold Niebuhr's guidance, whether you believe in a deity or not: "God grant me the serenity to accept the things I cannot change, courage to change the things I can, and wisdom to know the difference."

Takeaways

- Cortisol is a non-invasive window into your brain.

- HPA axis reprogramming due to early life stress leads to physical and psychological vulnerabilities.

- Cortisol is inversely related to happiness.[15]

- You can pass on a predisposition to stress to your kids and even your grandchildren through the reprogramming of the HPA axis.[16]

Chapter 4

Why Elite Athletes Measure Their Cortisol

Has a great athlete ever made you cry? We confess to weeping at the sight of the best tennis players slamming the winning serve, the strongest skaters landing a quadruple axel they worked a lifetime to master, the most sublime skiers putting down a triple like it's nothing.

When we knew we were going to work with Shadrack Kipchirchir, we got goosebumps. The distance track and field Olympian began partnering with us to monitor his cortisol levels so he could address overtraining — one of the most critical issues in competitive sports.

Don't turn the page if you're not a world-class athlete! Shadrack is a study in persistence, and every last one of us can learn from his story that it takes struggle to get where you want to go. From Shadrack — the runner and the man — we've learned that when your chin is on the ground, you pick yourself up, dust yourself off, and start all over again. Training for a race or any other long-term objective is about setting short- and long-term goals, and having the patience to overcome the inevitable setbacks. It's about preserving the sacred machine of body and mind you'll need to succeed in whatever competitive arena you choose.

Shadrack was used to winning. The Kenyan-born American runner had notched up titles in the Pan American Games, the World Championships in Athletics, and the USA Outdoor Track and Field Championships, where he won the cross-country crown in San Diego. But in his eleventh year as a competitive runner — right before the 2021 Olympic Trials in Tokyo — he tore a muscle in his left calf. The fact is, he wasn't completely surprised.

He'd begun to feel pain even while high-altitude training in Kenya. Shadrack had bought into the myth that a real athlete trains right through his pain.

As Bessel van der Kolk[1] puts it, the body keeps the score!

At Gate River Run in Jacksonville, Florida, Shadrack fell down a mile into a race and had to be carried off the field. He arranged to see a team of physicians and rehab specialists on the other side of the country at the Olympic Training Center in Colorado Springs, Colorado. On doctor's orders, he had to rest up for six weeks.

Bummed out doesn't begin to explain how he felt.

And the news only got worse. After six weeks, the tear had filled up with blood. He would need surgery. He informed his coach, manager, and Nike — his corporate sponsor — and expected to hear that, sadly, they couldn't support him anymore.

"But they supported me through the rehab process by constantly checking on me," Shadrack told Citius Mag, a track and field website.

Over the next ten months, Shadrack underwent rehab in Colorado. He was determined to heal and often showed up twice a day. His persistence paid off. In San Diego, Shadrack snatched victory from the jaws of defeat.

Shadrack Kipchirchir was in good hands. He had an experienced medical team, supportive coaches, knowledgeable trainers, and a loving wife about to give birth to their first child. He had what any competitive athlete could want.

Yet he knew he needed more. He needed to know what was happening inside his body and mind before he entered a competitive event. He went online to look for guidance. That's when he stumbled across some articles about cortisol and became acquainted with its role as the "messenger of stress." He wondered if he had over-trained and unwittingly put undue stress on his body and mind.

As a hormonal messenger, cortisol is involved in regulating essential functions in the body, including alertness, energy production and metabolism, blood pressure, blood-glucose levels, inflammation, and immune response. Additionally, cortisol is regulated by intricate feedback loops between the brain and adrenals.[2] Shadrack became increasingly convinced that cortisol was the biomarker to watch — more so than testosterone, heart-rate variability[3] (the amount of time between heartbeats), and Vo2 max (a measure of the minimum amount of oxygen the body can utilize during periods of increasing physical intensity). These other biomarkers vary little day by day, so that it's hard to rely on real-time information about changes in the body that athletes and their coaches need to know.

Indeed, research to date does not show any significant correlation between heart-rate variability (HRV), for example, and an athlete's physical recovery post-exertion. While more data need to be collected, cortisol in fact remains the most relevant biomarker for assessing whether it's safe for an athlete to train and compete.

We put the question to Dr. Maria Hopman, professor of integrative physiology at Radboud University Medical Center in Nijmegen, The Netherlands. Based on the research available today about recovery and readiness to train, do you think cortisol is a better biomarker for athletes than HRV?

True to her scientific integrity, Dr. Hopman is guarded but optimistic. "We don't yet have enough studies involving cortisol and hundreds of athletes," she says. "Before I come down in favor of one biomarker over another, I want to see more data. I need to see many measurement points before I reach any hard and fast conclusion. But I will give you a qualified yes. Cortisol is a better biomarker than HRV because it can change over a relatively short period of time. HRV doesn't. Testosterone doesn't.

WHY ELITE ATHLETES MEASURE THEIR CORTISOL

Vo2 max doesn't. If something doesn't change, how can you use it as a metric for anything?"

Shadrack is famous for running with a swinging movement of his right arm. He attributes his running style to a childhood habit of carrying his book bag over his left shoulder and propelling himself forward with his opposite arm.

All professional athletes develop habits that become their personal signature.[4] Likewise, stress is personal too. What bedevils one athlete may simply roll down the back of another.

Still, when athletes get together and compare stress, they discover certain commonalities.

One well-known study of track and field athletes participating in the 2015 European Games in Baku, Azerbaijan, for example, found that athletes tend to experience increased cortisol levels when they lose to other top athletes in their field.

At the same time, their stress level quantifiably increases when they defeat a fellow athlete they revere.

In short, losing hurts but winning can hurt too!

The Baku study also found that an increase in cortisol (and testosterone) before a competition may be detrimental to performance in track and field athletes.[5] Athletes with a less pronounced endocrine response in the 24 hours before an important competition fared better than those exhibiting greater endocrine changes.

Because so much about cortisol can be contradictory, Shadrack wanted more actionable advice. Once he was on the mend, he committed himself to understand what had led to the tear in his calf muscle — and what he could do to avoid injuring himself again. When we met in Colorado Springs, our teams set him up with a rapid salivary cortisol test during his race week.

First, we established Shadrack's baseline cortisol rhythm by measuring his levels five times on January 6. A baseline would help us understand his average cortisol rhythm and let us identify any outlier stress during competition week. This first step was critical. Just as Shadrack has his own way of running, he also has cortisol levels unique to him. Everyone's baseline is different because everyone's sleep-wake cycle, exercise regimen, diet, and overall health are different. We needed to understand how cortisol normally behaved in Shadrack's body so we could compare his cortisol levels the day before, the day of, and the day after the race.

Here's what Shadrack's baseline cortisol levels looked like. Note the relatively high cortisol awakening response at 7:15 a.m.

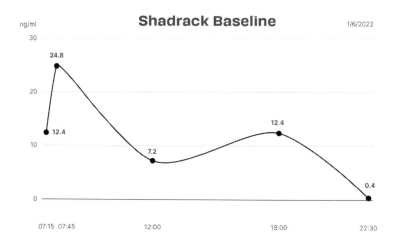

Now let's look at Shadrack's morning and evening measurements from January 6 to 10 — two days before the race (January 6), the day of the race (January 8), and two days after (January 10). You'll observe that Shadrack's cortisol levels are relatively high on the day after the race, a likely sign that his body is still recovering from inflammation and muscle fatigue.

WHY ELITE ATHLETES MEASURE THEIR CORTISOL

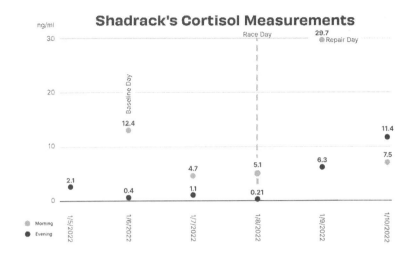

And here are Shadrack's morning measurements for January and February.

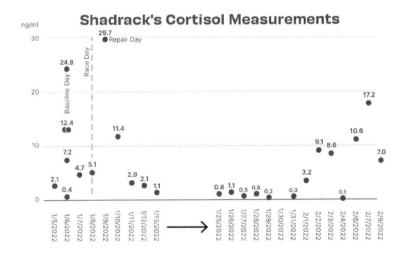

Shadrack's baseline on January 6 — two days before the race — shows that his scores are prone to extremes. He scored 24.8 at his peak — dramatically higher than a more typical 6 for nonathletes. And he saw another jump later in the day to around 12.4, when his cortisol levels should have been steadily declining. What might this say about his performance readiness?

We hypothesized that Shadrack was already stressed on January 6, thirty minutes after waking up. We ruled out physical stress. Shadrack's training load had been tapering off in the days right before the race.

We also took into account that this was Shadrack's first competition in 294 days. Being human, he had personal stresses to think about in addition to the race. Those might have contributed to his high 24.8 cortisol reading.

A level of 24.8 would be a red flag for a non-athlete, especially if that number didn't come down quickly. For a competitive runner like Shadrack, cortisol levels can bounce high and low.

At 1:00 p.m on January 8, the day of the race, Shadrack came in first place.

At 8 p.m., the same day, we noticed Shadrack's cortisol was extremely low (approximately 0.2). We were baffled — and concerned. We had expected to see a stark rise in the hormone typical of physical stress immediately after the race, with a gradual drop for the evening. Eight hours after the race, we expected that the spike in cortisol would have been resolved. We contemplated two possibilities. Either the measurement reflected an inaccurate reading, or Shadrack was showing signs of burnout. His massive exertion could have temporarily exhausted his body.

On January 9, Shadrack's wake-up cortisol level was 29.7. That's super-high. Shouldn't his cortisol have subsided? After all, he won the race. What was stressing him out? We can attest he wasn't upset after besting his competition, as the Baku study in Nature Journal observed in the case of some runners![6]

Our experts speculated that Shadrack was recovering from the wear and tear his body suffered during his extreme exertion.

All good interpretations. Over time we'll have additional

granular data to give us a more nuanced look at the impact of stress on Shadrack's body.

We hope other competitive athletes start monitoring their cortisol levels, especially as many openly admit to dealing with the consequences of physical or emotional stress. We want to see female athletes start monitoring their cortisol levels, especially because their hormone levels vary cyclically.[7] Would a seasoned tennis player like Simona Halep, for example, ranked Number 1 in singles twice between 2017 and 2019 for a total of 64 weeks, have succumbed to a panic attack in her thirteenth French Open while playing 19-year-old Zheng Qinwen if she had been aware of her body's biochemistry? Would Naomi Osaka have withdrawn from her French Open if she had understood the probable connection between her cortisol levels and the depression she felt after defeating Serena Williams — her tennis idol? Could Simone Biles, one of the world's most breathtaking gymnasts, have averted her various training-related injuries by monitoring her cortisol levels?

Data show that some 35 percent of elite athletes suffer from stress, eating disorders, body image issues, burnout, suicidal thoughts, depression, panic attacks, or anxiety. All honor Olympic swimmer Michael Phelps, USC volleyball player Victoria Garrick, and NBA player Kevin Love for speaking frankly about their own mental health struggles. Just more reason to respect and admire these "GOAT" athletes — the "greatest of all time." We believe cortisol monitoring can aid in their self-care too.

———

A lot of athletes are starting to ask themselves, "Is winning supposed to feel this bad?"

Clinical psychologist Alia Crum, who has spent years

studying mindset at Stanford's Mind & Body Lab, takes a nuanced view of the body's natural response to stress.

"Cortisol was not designed to kill us," she says. "It was designed to boost our cognitive functioning, narrow our attention, and activate our bodies in ways that help us meet the demands we're faced with."

Crum asserts that the negative side of stress is only one side of the coin. "We need to be aware of the positive effects of stress and realize that having the right mindset will help us shape our response to stress in a way that can help us win a race or achieve any other competitive goal."

Crum and her Stanford colleagues devised an experiment to demonstrate how an affirmative mindset can help individuals cope with a high-stress situation.

For a typical morning class of 100 university students, Crum and her research team measured the students' cortisol levels. Doing so, she was able to get a baseline reading for each individual.

At a later date, the same students attended a class in which a Stanford Graduate School of Business professor led a lecture-workshop on charisma. Then students had ten minutes to prepare a speech — an activity meant to simulate a stressful situation. When the ten minutes were up, the professor randomly chose five people to stand before the class, give the speech, and have the other students evaluate them on their charisma. Using a salivary test, Crum measured the students' cortisol levels after they finished dashing off their speeches.

"The students tended to take on two different profiles," Professor Crum told us. "One group of students freaked out, and we were not surprised to see a rise in their cortisol levels. The other group seemed to be sort of disengaged from the task. Their cortisol levels hadn't moved much, and in some cases, they were lower. Now, neither freaking out nor being disengaged is an adaptive way to approach a stressful task. What's adaptive is to be appropriately engaged — to be physiologically aroused to meet the demand. We found that the truly adaptive response was a moderate level of cortisol elevation. The students who had a 'stress is enhancing' mindset were more likely to be in this desired middle range of cortisol response. By contrast, neither the freaked out nor the disengaged individuals had an appropriate response."

When it comes to stress — in the classroom or the running track — the most adaptive approach to a challenge harkens back to our Goldilocks principle: You want your porridge just right: Not too hot, not too cold.

When it comes to pressure-cooker sports, you want a mindset that's just right enough to incite your inner competitive beast without destroying your sense of self.

More easily said than done, right?

Yet, in Shadrack, we have an example of a competitive athlete who has done just that.

"When I came to the United States to study engineering at Western Kentucky University and Oklahoma State University, I thought of myself as a student athlete, not an athlete-student," he said. "I was attentive to my cross-country running, but I knew I had to take care of my academics first."

Balance. A time and place for everything.

Despite his drive to win, Shadrack was also pulled in another life-changing direction. When he witnessed how the U.S. Army had turned his two "playboy" brothers into mature young men, Shadrack enlisted too.

He had no intention of abandoning his running career, and in the Army he joined its World Class Athlete Program. One year later, he finished fourth in the Pan American Games' 10,000 meter race. The World Championships in Athletics, the Summer Olympics, the USA Cross Country Championships, and sponsorship by Nike followed.

"I have tried to connect my running ambitions with a higher mission," Shadrack told us. "Duty called. I wanted to serve."

Shadrack's decision brought out an army of critics.

"The naysayers didn't affect me at all," he said. "At the end of the day, it was my decision to do what was right for my country, my family, and myself."

But Shadrack! A training moratorium from June until November! What could the Army offer you but push-ups and sit-ups, day in, day out!

Shadrack resumed his competitive training schedule right after boot camp.

He insists he doesn't have a silver bullet, but in working with him, we've come to believe that more American and European athletes would benefit from taking a page from his playbook. We've rarely seen an athletic mindset as thoughtful, measured, and modest as Shadrack's. He strikes us as perfectly in sync with Ali Crum's mindset philosophy when she says, "We can influence the way our body responds in part by changing our mindset."

"I have my engineering degrees, and one day — after I exhaust my poor hamstrings — I will pursue engineering work," he said.

An intelligent plan.

In the meantime, Shadrack will measure his cortisol levels every day and literally stay on track. He'll know when his cortisol levels are super-high, and he might decide to wait until they come down a bit before setting out for the track.

And we're going to help him keep those poor hamstrings strong — until he runs to meet the next phase of his life.

Takeaways

- Cortisol is the No.1 marker of athletic recovery.

- Knowing your cortisol levels can help athletes limit their injuries and optimize their training.[8]

- Mindset affects the way an athlete's body responds to mental and physical stress.[9]

Chapter 5

Stress, Infertility, and Cortisol

Everyone's heard about the couple who tried for years to get pregnant and finally succeeded only after adopting a baby. The popular wisdom goes that conception will definitely happen if the woman only "relaxes." You can imagine how relaxing it is to hear, "Just relax! You'll be pregnant in no time."

If only it were that simple.

While research on this adoption-then-pregnancy scenario is still underway, we are nonetheless prepared to say there's mounting evidence that stress, and accompanying high cortisol levels, are causing infertility. And if you could return your cortisol levels to what's normal for you, you'd remove at least one obstacle in the way of you getting pregnant.

If you've been trying to get pregnant and you haven't conceived yet, you'll want to read on. We won't insult your intelligence with a sermon about having the right mindset, and certainly won't advise you to start an adoption process as a way of reeling in a baby.

Some 15% to 30% of couples will be diagnosed with unexplained infertility after their diagnostic workup.[1] These figures are alarming and, sadly, they represent a long-time downward trend. In fact, from 1960 to 2018, the total fertility rate worldwide has dropped by 1% a year.[2] This might not sound like much, but the numbers add up to more than 10% per decade and more than 50% over 50 years. . A headline in *The Irish Examiner* foretells a dystopic future we find terrifying to contemplate: " Most couples may need to use IVF by 2050: Are we facing spermageddon?"

By now you know our position: Elevated levels of cortisol —

the biological manifestation of stress — are behind disease of nearly every kind. Infertility is no exception.

When you're in a state of chronic stress, glucocorticoids — cholesterol-derived steroid hormones produced in the outer cortex of the adrenal gland — are released into the blood. Under normal conditions, glucocorticoids regulate many cellular functions, including metabolism, cognition, inflammation, cell development and homeostasis. In times of stress, however, if the body occupies "fight or flight" mode, a rise in glucocorticoids suppresses the reproductive functions of the hypothalamic-pituitary-gonadal (HPG) axis — the complex processing center that coordinates an assembly line of sex hormones in both sexes.

For women in stressful situations, high cortisol levels inhibit the expression of gonadotropin-releasing hormone (GnHR), the hormone that causes the pituitary gland in the brain to make and secrete luteinizing hormone (LH) and follicle-stimulating hormone (FSH). When your body is in a balanced state, LH and FSH stimulate the ovaries to make estrogen and progesterone. But with stress on the body from depression, malnutrition, infection, or anxiety, for example, the feedback loops that keep the HPG axis and its HPA partner axis humming along, are interrupted. And since making cortisol for survival is perceived by the body as a priority, sex hormone production is diminished or thwarted altogether.

What we've offered here is a thumbnail sketch of the biochemical cascade your body produces in the face of psychological or physiological stresses. The mechanisms of the HPA-HPG axes are enormously intricate, alternately involving the stimulation and inhibition of hormone production. Suffice it to say that when these mechanisms are thrown off-kilter, getting pregnant is virtually impossible.

Chronic inflammation — one such consequence of HPA-HPG malfunction — can affect ovulation, hormone production, and implantation of a fertilized egg in the uterus. As researchers have learned, embryo implantation requires a series of well-coordinated events, regulated by estrogen and progesterone, but remember, abnormal cortisol has the loudest voice. You owe it to yourself to try a more holistic approach before undergoing any chemical intervention or in vitro fertilization.

In your quest to turn your infertility into fertility, take one day at a time.

We are finely tuned beings, and it doesn't take all that much stress to knock the HPA-HPG axes off kilter.

Sarah L. Berga MD, a reproductive endocrinology professor at the Jacobs School of Medicine and Biomedical Sciences, SUNY, Buffalo, was part of a team that studied healthy women, termed the "walking well," who were nonetheless amenorrheic – that is, suffering from an abnormal absence of menstruation. To all outer appearances, the women were physically fit. Berga wanted to understand what was happening to them at the neuroendocrine level.

She and her team designed a monkey model in which they gave the monkeys two kinds of stressors. One was an energy stressor where the monkeys, now on a 20% reduced diet, ran two miles a day on a treadmill.[3] "The monkeys actually liked the treadmill," Berga says. "We had to bribe them to get off because, like most human runners, they liked it."

The second stressor involved moving the monkeys' cages around. They now had new neighbors all the time. "Imagine that you had to go to a new hotel room every day," Berga says. "It would be kind of stressful, but in the scheme of things, it would be a relatively mild stress."

Berga and her team observed that when the monkeys were given just one of the two stressors, they were fine. "But when we imposed both of the stressors on them, 70% of the monkeys had transient loss of ovulatory function," she says. "And that's what was happening to our humans. A little of this and a little of that – and suddenly you have the perfect storm for chronic stress. Even everyday, low magnitude amount of stress makes you feel out of control. What do you do? You eat less. You exercise a little more to feel as if you are 'doing something.' And still your cortisol levels are high."

It's stunning. The women, who experienced what we think of as the normal stresses of everyday life, were amenorrheic by dint of a modest increase of cortisol at night.

Just as stunning is Berga's solution.

"We didn't tell the women to eat less," she says. "We didn't tell them to exercise more. We tried to help them figure out what makes them feel like they're in control. Mysteriously, or should I say, with some cognitive behavioral therapy, their cortisol gets better at night – and they start to ovulate."[4]

In a separate human study, Berga and her team recruited women with amenorrhea (abnormal ovulation) and eumenorrhea (normal ovulation) to see if cortisol levels in their cerebrospinal fluid (CSF) were comparable. All the women had normal body weight. Blood samples were collected at 15-minute intervals for 24 hours, followed by 25 ml draws of cerebrospinal fluid. The results: Cortisol concentrations in the CSF were 30% greater when serum (blood) cortisol was 16% higher in the amenorrheic women compared with eumenorrheic women. Berga's conclusion: The HPA axis is activated in the amenorrheic women. The normal feedback mechanisms are perturbed and cortisol levels remain high. This study was the first to associate CSF cortisol with "reproductive compromise."[5]

The takeaway here, Berga says, is that cortisol is a master hormone. "The concept I'm building is a U-shaped curve, and in the case of cortisol, the 'U' is very narrow," she says. "A little too much, a little too little, and suddenly you are in trouble physiologically. It's not a profound change, and historically, it hasn't been easy to measure."

In fact, as Berga argues, physicians used to measure a single time period of cortisol activity and could infer, mistakenly, that body functions were normal.

"Actually, they weren't normal," Berga says. "The problem was we used to measure a single time point and then didn't consider how cortisol was interacting with other hormones or chemicals in the body. For example, let's say somebody is in a motor vehicle accident and they injure their pituitary stalk. The first two hormones we need to replace are cortisol and thyroid. If you replace one without the other, you will kill the patient."

Figure 1

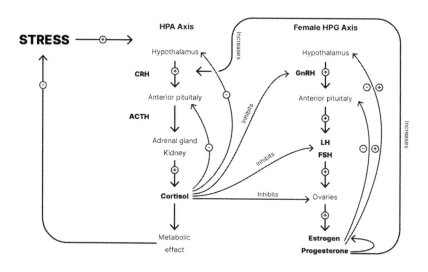

Here's a schematic of what happens when cortisol overrides the entire reproductive (and immune) systems in our bodies.

What the body wants, Berga says, is homeostasis. "When all of your 'U's' are at the right level, everything is interconnected hypothalamically, and everything works fine," she says. "The master signals are neural, and they cascade down into this

STRESS, INFERTILITY, AND CORTISOL

exquisite machinery that I view with reverence. If you need a little extra cortisol to step up your game in the face of chronic stress, the body will give it to you. But that super-boost of cortisol is not going to be great for your reproduction. The body makes a tradeoff."

———

We need to look at another side of infertility: The absence of functional sperm in the male partner.

The male factor is the sole or contributing cause in about one-half of infertility cases. Indeed, some studies have found a negative correlation between cortisol and libido, testosterone production and sperm motility to enumerate a few. The "progressive motility" of sperm — and sperm speed is a significant predictor of the woman's chance of getting pregnant. Put another way, an influx of cortisol puts a ball and chain on testosterone and sperm, and they slow down. Before seeking medical attention, men must take an honest look at what they can do to produce healthy sperm. There's actually something pretty simple you can do: Think about the food you put in your mouth. Are you avoiding good fats? Don't! Sperm will thrive if you follow a high-fat, low-carb diet of beef, liver, salmon, sardines, tuna, oysters, pork, Brazil nuts, walnuts, tomatoes, and garlic. In combination, these foods supply sperm with L-carnitine, coenzyme Q10, Vitamin C, Vitamin E, selenium, and omega 3's. This is a rich enough list that will satisfy most carnivores and vegetarians.

Changing habits is not like changing your socks. Admittedly, it'll be hard. Once again — take one day at a time. Your palate probably acquired its taste for chips, pretzels, danish and fried foods in childhood, and a more wholesome, more mature diet could take getting used to. One day at a time.

We'd like to recommend the salmon grilled with honey and

mustard, mashed potatoes with butter and milk, and sauerkraut. Delicious.

Let's say you've already conferred with your OB-GYN and she has already started you on a particular infertility treatment regimen. Will your anxiety about the treatment, or your constant thinking about it, throw your cortisol levels into chronic high gear — and therefore undermine the therapy? Maybe it'd be better not to think about infertility or pregnancy at all. Just decide, "I'm done thinking about this!"

Not the way to go. As with most problems, including infertility, avoidance is a terrible solution.

A 2021 study revealed that women who avoided thinking about infertility or their infertility therapy have higher stress scores and lower quality of life. Turns out that "active avoidance coping," or pretending stressors don't really exist, may undermine treatment associated with generally good therapeutic results. And no surprise here: Female study participants who used active avoidance coping as a coping strategy — or anti-strategy — had elevated cortisol levels.

Anyone who's tried to improve their outlook on life knows how hard it is to break self-defeating mental habits. Polish fertility researchers in 2019 wanted to analyze the stigma associated with fertility problems and the reluctance by Polish couples to seek support from family or friends. In Stage 1 of the experimental study, saliva samples were taken from the participants to ascertain cortisol levels. In Stage 2, a control group viewed an informational video about human embryology, and an experimental group underwent a process of "supportive social interaction." In Stage 3 all study participants had their cortisol levels checked again. A statistical analysis of the results pointed to a significant decrease in stress — and in cortisol levels — in the group receiving social support.

In short, evidence supported the study's hypothesis that social support during fertility treatment significantly lowered stress and cortisol levels. Moreover, the researchers found that all kinds of social support, including partner-to-partner support, institutional support (individual or couples therapy), and informal support groups helped lower stress and cortisol in women undergoing infertility treatment. Stress and cortisol levels in men dropped too if they felt emotionally supported.

However rewarding your work is, you probably have to deal with deadlines, sales targets, and ornery colleagues. Have you considered the possibility that your workplace is stressing you out — and that you spend an unnecessary amount of time in it?

As self-proclaimed busy bees, we are sensitive to allegations that we put in too many hours at the office. We're both driven personalities, whose sense of self hinges on the mark we want to make in our respective professions. For ourselves, and for our workaholic brethren, it's our duty to ask, "Is our workload contributing to our stress, and ultimately, to our high levels of cortisol?" If you are in your twenties, thirties, or early forties, you might be prone to infertility based almost solely on the high-stress work you do and love.

Female doctors, for example, have unique challenges when they decide to get pregnant. One such study in 2012-2013 of 600 female physicians who graduated medical school between 1995 and 2000 found that nearly one-quarter of respondents trying to conceive was diagnosed with infertility, double the infertility rate in the general population.[6]. The researchers concluded that for a substantial proportion of female physicians, combining a medical career with motherhood poses challenges.

Another study surveying pregnancy and fertility trends among female otolaryngologists found that almost one-third of respondents — mean age of 32.3 — who attempted to conceive were diagnosed with infertility.

Women in other lines of work, from law to agriculture, have experienced infertility too, as have women with jobs that involve heavy lifting. In this latter category, women who worked evening or nighttime shifts had fewer mature eggs than women whose jobs did not involve heavy lifting or work during the same hours.

We're the last people in the world to tell you to dampen your career ambitions. But forewarned is forearmed. The more you know about the relationship between stress, cortisol and infertility, the better equipped you'll be to map out a career and a family life.

Gentlemen, we're talking to you too! You also need to be mindful of your reproductive health.

Another Polish study,[7] assessing the effect of stress on semen quality, revealed that stressful situations at work have a negative impact on semen volume and percent of "progressive spermatozoa," or, the ability of sperm to move efficiently.[8]

A comparable Israeli study[9] found that prolonged stress, as in soldiers on active wartime duty, reduced sperm quality. Researchers at Rutgers School of Public Health and Columbia University's Mailman School of Public Health have confirmed the correlations observed in both the Polish and Israeli studies.

We'd be untrue to ourselves if we told men to seek out careers in placid workplaces (do such places exist?), and arrogant if we told them to avoid living in geopolitically insecure zones. All we can do is offer men the advice we offer women: Be aware that stress may affect your reproductive ability. And know you can mitigate the stress that's part of life in a society that promises career satisfaction — at a cost.

STRESS, INFERTILITY, AND CORTISOL

If you don't get pregnant as fast as you'd like, your first stop should be your OB-GYN's office. Any number of physiological or lifestyle factors can impact fertility. Among them: Elderly primigravida (first pregnancy at age 35 or older); diabetes; eating disorders; excessive alcohol consumption or drug abuse; exposure to environmental toxins; over-exercising; sexually transmitted diseases; smoking; obesity; thyroid disease; celiac disease, kidney disease; or sickle cell anemia. A lot can go wrong with the human body, and only a medical professional can diagnose the source of infertility in women and men. We advocate testing, not guessing.

Meanwhile, you can take action to put your body into reproduction mode by following the advice in our mindset and recommendations chapters.

If we stress monkeys want to have some little primates in our lives, we have to . . . relax. But relax intelligently. Our bodies are smart. When you show yourself some love, your body will love you back. After all, when your reproductive function grinds to a halt, your body is asking you to take better care of your whole self. It tells you that if you're swimming in stress, it cannot allot resources to making a baby. It's marshaling those resources to keep you alive.

Let's take a tip from our own HPA-HPG axes. They want to stay in balance with each other. Likewise, we need to be in balance with our environment. If you accept that the human body is a magnificently calibrated machine, you'll respect its capacities and its limitations. We don't live forever. Let's work with nature, not against it.

Takeaways

- Elevated cortisol levels are probably the #1 overlooked cause of infertility.

CORTISOL: THE MASTER HORMONE

- A cortisol increase of as little as 20% in the morning can stop ovulation, rendering any woman infertile, and is probably the No. 1 cause of unexplained infertility. Normalizing cortisol levels has helped women get pregnant.[10,11]

- Men's testosterone levels and sperm quality go down as a result of elevated cortisol.[12,13]

Chapter 6

Stress, Menopause, and Cortisol

Gentlemen! Don't skip this chapter. If you've got a woman in your life, you'll want to understand what's happening to her, body and mind, as she enters perimenopause and menopause.

News headlines about women reflect an all too familiar social and psychological reality:

"Workplace Stress Hits Women Harder than Men"

"Why the 'Sandwich Generation' Is So Stressed Out"

"Money, Job Stress Continue to Weigh on Women"

Women in the developed world have so many material advantages compared to women in developing or war-torn countries, but they are also far more likely to deal with the many consequences of a high-tech, high-stress society. Our foremothers campaigned so hard for our right to vote, our right to set career goals and achieve them, our right to healthcare, that we tell ourselves, "No problem. I can deal with everything."

Our bodies tell us we really can't. Nobody, men included, can handle an onslaught of emotional, vocational, and financial pressures without succumbing to chronic pain, depression, sadness, exhaustion, weight gain, inflammation — sadly, the list of adverse stress-related effects goes on and on. And women don't get a free pass. In all too many places, they cope with war, sexual violence, famine, limited educational options and lack of potable water every day.

Living in a competitive, high-tech, consumer-driven society exacts a unique toll on us. Indeed, the environmental burdens we bear can be so intractable that Bruce McEwen introduced the concept of "allostatic load" in 1993 to describe the price we pay for chronic exposure to the heightened physiological responses we endure in an environment full of normal and over-the-top stress. These include the consequences of health-damaging behaviors such as poor sleep and circadian disruption, lack of exercise, smoking, alcohol consumption, and unhealthy diet. When environmental challenges overwhelm us, allostatic overload occurs as the body transitions to a state where the stress response systems are activated repeatedly and buffering factors are not adequate.[1]

It's a paradox: The systems that react to stress — the autonomic nervous system and HPA axis system— protect us in the short run. But when stress is unremitting, it causes damage or disease.

Rich or poor, physically safe or under threat, the price we pay for overstimulating our bodily systems ultimately results in what neuroscientist Bruce McEwen in 1993 termed "allostatic load."[2] It's when this allostatic load — the wear and tear of daily life on the body over long periods of time — becomes too heavy that it leads to disease.

Because stress is both cumulative and additive, we women can move mountains, but we cannot ignore the strain of chronic stress on our bodies.

As we saw in Chapter 2, "Why You Should Measure Your Cortisol Levels," the onset of stress provokes a cascade of biochemical events in the body, starting with the hypothalamic-pituitary-adrenal axis (HPA). To recap, the HPA axis is a complex system of neuroendocrine pathways and feedback loops that work to maintain homeostasis, the process by which the body achieves stability in a world of ever-changing conditions. The HPA axis is the frontline worker in the body's confrontation with stress.

When women (and men) are not stressed, the HPA and HPG axes are a compatible couple. But when people are stressed —

when their allostatic load is heavy — their HPA and HPG axes are out of kilter with each other. At the hypothalamic level (the "H" in HPA), the stressor activates the corticotropin-released hormone (CRH) and arginine vasopressin (AVP). These hormones stimulate the anterior lobe of the pituitary gland, which releases adrenocorticotropic hormone (ACTH), which in turn stimulates the synthesis of cortisol. If stress remains constant, the HPA enters a state of "dysregulation." Soon any number of systems, suddenly awash in cortisol, go haywire. The HPG axis comes to a standstill and HPT (Hypothalamic-Pituitary-Thyroid axis) slows down.

For better or worse, this biochemical "perfect storm" is almost inevitable as women enter perimenopause, the runway to menopause. Estrogens start to drastically fall off, after severe fluctuation during premenopause, for a few months to about a year.[3] Twelve months after our last menstrual period, our estrogen and progesterone-producing factory in the ovaries shut down and we are in full-blown menopause.

Any time a woman experiences fluctuations of estrogen and progesterone, her body is in stress. And, wow, is the body ever in distress during its "midlife crisis." Even in the best of times you don't want to stress the adrenal gland because it will overproduce cortisol — and your body will make even less of the estrogen and progesterone it needs to stay in balance. That's a difficult menopause in a nutshell: under stress, while protective and nourishing estrogens and progesterone drop, cortisol goes haywire, making everything much worse if you're not careful.

Let's look more closely at the physiological theater stress enacts at midlife — and how we experience this "performance" throughout our bodies.

When a (real or perceived) stressful incident occurs, our

sympathetic nervous system releases epinephrine (adrenaline) and norepinephrine (noradrenaline) within seconds. The former increases cardiac output and raises glucose levels in the blood. The latter increases the force of skeletal muscle contraction and the rate and force of heart contractions.

Within seconds, the HPA axis also gets the message: we need cortisol. The hypothalamus (the "H" of HPA) responds to elevated norepinephrine levels by secreting corticotropin-releasing hormone (CRH) into the bloodstream. CRH also revs up the sympathetic nervous system and further exacerbates heart rate.

At the same time, CRH tells the pituitary gland (the "P" of HPA) to release adrenocorticotropic hormone (ACTH) into the bloodstream. ACTH travels through the bloodstream to the adrenal glands, specifically the outer layer, or adrenal cortex. ACTH binds to receptors on the surface of the adrenal cortex. The result is a series of intracellular events that compel the adrenal glands to secrete glucocorticoids such as cortisol in humans.

In fight-or-flight situations, cortisol helps us survive: It increases blood pressure and heart rate, and provides more blood to skeletal muscles so we can flee or fight back. It also expedites the circulation of glucose in our blood to help our body's cells ramp up energy. Normally, the danger passes and all should calm down.

But during menopause, and the perimenopausal lead-up to it, elevated cortisol coincides with severe symptoms, such as seven or more hot flashes a day, anxiety, depression, and lack of sexual desire. The "change of life" may be part of nature's plan, but, in the presence of elevated cortisol, our bodies respond to it as an unwelcome intruder.

Indeed, when cortisol levels rise during menopause, we feel emotionally stressed because our bodies experience stress at the glandular level. The ovaries, for example, start to close up shop at perimenopause. If they could speak, they would say, "I'm tired. I don't want to produce hormones anymore." By full-fledged menopause, the ovaries produce virtually no estrogen and progesterone — the hormones that biologically define the female of the human species.

Before menopause hits, cortisol is higher in the morning because we need a stimulus to wake us up. Cortisol levels subside throughout the day, leveling off toward nightfall, so we can fall asleep. With stress and the approach to menopause though, cortisol levels surge throughout the day. With each spike in levels, our body rapidly releases more sugar in the blood. Blood pressure rises because our body needs more energy to deal with this barrage of menopausal symptoms. With so much cortisol swirling through our bodies, a good night's sleep is more dream than reality. And the antidote for interrupted sleep — progesterone — is produced at much lower quantities and by the already stressed adrenal glands.

Our bodies do not take these changes lightly. Research studies increasingly indicate a strong relationship in menopause between elevated cortisol levels and major depression, lower bone density and cognitive complaints.[4,5] Women in late perimenopause have exhibited higher total cholesterol and LDL-cholesterol (the "bad cholesterol"). Ultimately, large shifts in cortisol levels unopposed by the nourishing, building support of estrogens and testosterone at a woman's mid-life, may be increasing the risk of metabolic syndrome - we become vulnerable to hyperlipidemia, heart disease, obesity, stroke and type 2 diabetes.

A word about muscles. To stay strong and independent into old age, we need to have and keep enough muscle mass. You wouldn't guess it, but loss of muscle mass has been associated with cognitive decline in elderly.[6] As menopause hits and the testosterone levels drop, if your cortisol is elevated you will break down more muscle. There is no better time to lift weights than menopause, ladies! To build and maintain your muscles, you need to eat enough good quality protein and lift heavy weights. Caveat: wrong type of exercise - too intense or too prolonged - will raise your cortisol and lead to muscle loss and higher body fat percentage. Join a class[7] or find a personal trainer who understands that you should not exercise like a 20 year old man. Extra good news: your bones will get stronger and you can have another yummy treat without the guilt - your muscles will gobble it.

Some studies have also shown that high cortisol levels in menopausal women result in decreased brain volume. Consequently, some women experience mental fog, depression or anxiety.

Forestalling the most severe effects of menopause requires a recommitment to your overall health. Here is what you can do to manage — even subvert — some of the most unpleasant menopausal symptoms:

First, embrace an optimistic mindset. Accept the challenge in your late forties and early fifties that your body will undergo significant changes — and that you can mitigate the impact of this biochemical tsunami. Positive mindsets are not inconsequential, according to Stanford Mind and Body Lab investigator Dr. Alia Crum. "They play a dramatic role in determining our health and well-being," as she told a TEDx gathering in 2014.

Can a "mind over matter" outlook really help us deal with menopause?

Definitely.

Mind over matter, or the non-chemical healing properties of the placebo effect, is no fantasy. The issue is not whether menopause-related stress is good or bad. It's whether we are ready to acknowledge the stress and turn it to our advantage.

Menopause can be tough going, but it offers us an opportunity to take stock of our health. We can even use menopause to acquire wisdom and achieve personal growth.

First, you want to pay attention to:

- Weight gain, especially in your abdomen and face
- Muscle weakness and volume loss in your thighs and arms
- Interrupted sleep

Second, you need to notice what's going on with your heart and mind. Among the most common emotional symptoms during perimenopause and menopause: irritability, feelings of sadness, lack of motivation, anxiety, aggressiveness, difficulty concentrating, fatigue, and moodiness.

Third, you'll want to measure your cortisol levels and correct them.

Fourth, get more muscles and exercise the right way.

In an era where "there's an app for that," salivary testing puts cortisol measurement in your own hands. You'll want to establish a baseline understanding of your cortisol level by checking it five times on Day One at regular intervals. (You and your healthcare provider may decide to take measurements on a daily, weekly, or monthly basis.) You can see your numeric results almost instantaneously and share them with your physician.

Knowing your cortisol levels will help you take action to bring your HPA axis into equilibrium and help your adrenal glands better cope with their menopausal extra duties.

Takeaways

- Chronically high cortisol levels exacerbate menopausal symptoms.

- Cortisol is probably one of the most important causes of your sleep issues, mood changes, and depression.

- Changes in cortisol patterns affect energy, sleep, weight, mood and longevity.[8]

- The negative effects of elevated cortisol are amplified in menopausal women by lack of compensatory anabolic hormones like estrogens, testosterone and DHEA. The result: unfavorable body composition changes with muscle and bone loss, and gain of visceral fat.

- Keep your muscles to stay strong, smart and independent - by eating enough good quality protein and exercising the right way to avoid raising cortisol.

Chapter 7

What's the Gut and the Microbiome Got to Do with Cortisol?

Want to hear something wild? Researchers who study the gut microbiome — the intricate community of bacteria, viruses, and yeast in your gut — connect it to the health of our sex hormones. A higher abundance of *Bacteroidetes* and a lower abundance of *Firmicutes*, for example, produce higher estrogen levels in healthy women. And that, depending on your genetic make-up, is not always a good thing. In healthy men, *Ruminococcus* and *Acinetobacter* appear to raise testosterone levels. Indeed, the microbiome, whose microbes account for as much as five pounds of our body weight, regulates our endocrine systems and influences hormone behavior. As with the HPA and HPG axes,[1] the relationship between the microbiome and our hormones is flexible and bi-directional: Hormones affect the diversity of our gut microbiome, and our gut microbiome influences hormone production and functionality. While much research still needs to be done, we're learning that the gut microbiome plays an important role in shaping brain function and behavior, including the activity of the HPA and HPG axes.[2]

No system in the body is an island. The hip bone's connected to the thigh bone, right? That's also the case with the brain: It's connected to the gut via a "north-south" highway called the gut-brain axis. Sure enough, researchers in the College of Agricultural, Consumer and Environmental Sciences at the University of Illinois found that cortisol in the gut-brain axis facilitates the relationship between the "good" bacterium *Ruminococcus* and an essential amino acid in the brain called n-acetylaspartate, or

NAA. Interactions, such as this one between the gut "microbiota" and the brain, are happening all the time.

Wait! Isn't cortisol often a problem in our bodies?

No. At least not when it's doing what it's great at doing. As we've suggested, we members of *homo sapiens* would never have gotten this far if we didn't have cortisol — the stress hormone — to alert us to physical danger or unhealthy psychological provocation, and to get us ready for the day in the morning. Cortisol is our higher power! When we've got the right amount of it at the right time, our bodies experience homeostasis. In fact, when we have too little, we're in big trouble. The result is fatigue, unintentional weight loss, low blood sugar, sugar and salt cravings, low blood pressure and dizziness, to name a few. At the extreme, we suffer from a condition called "adrenal insufficiency," or Addison's Disease and that, under stress, can be fatal.

In fact, other conditions are characterized by low cortisol levels, including rheumatoid arthritis, asthma, chronic fatigue syndrome, and lupus. William McK. Jefferies,[3] a physician who for decades has advocated the safe uses of cortisol in small, physiologic doses, has had excellent results with women who originally presented with infertility. Dr. Jefferies has called cortisol "one of the most promising therapeutic agents of all time," but noted that, if an excessive amount of glucocorticoids are present or given before a challenge to the immune system, this will interfere or block the HPA response with disastrous results.

The same follows for cortisol and the gut. As a facilitator of the gut-brain axis, cortisol is good indeed. But when cortisol levels are out of balance, all hell breaks loose both in the gut microbiome and at the gut wall lining.

These microbes are listening in on the conversation between your brain and gut and will cut in, interfering with the response sent back to the brain. As such, the interplay between your microbiome and your brain affects not only the health of your sex hormones, but also your mental health, brain development, cognition, social behavior and neuroinflammation — the activation of the brain's innate immune system in response to any inflammatory stimulus.

How stress, and by implication, cortisol, affects the microbiome is not yet completely understood, but we have known for over 80 years[4] that stress results in swollen adrenal glands (our stress hormones maker), shrunken thymus (our immune training center) and stomach ulcers. Indeed, we need the right amount of cortisol to initiate a controlled inflammatory and immune response in order to repair tissues. Recent studies have also found that elevated cortisol levels may lead to an unhealthy increase in opportunistic pathogens, or disease-causing microbes resulting in dysbiosis. If you think that cortisol is the usual suspect, you're right — and wrong! Glucocorticoids, i.e. cortisol in humans, exert both stimulatory *and* inhibitory effects on certain gut microbes and their metabolites. Moreover, our own stress influences the microbiome, and the microbiome influences our body's response. Microbiota and their metabolites[5] are known to exert effects throughout the HPA axis, influencing glucocorticoid synthesis, release and signaling pathways. And we're back where we started![6]

Let's go back to the beginning of human life.

As you've seen in Chapter 5 ("Stress, Infertility, and Cortisol"), pregnancy is unlikely to occur when the HPA-HPG axes are not working in concert with each other — and elevated cortisol is oftentimes the number one cause here.[7] Growing evidence also suggests that stress, which results in cortisol elevation, has an impact on the relationship between the gut microbiome and estrogens. A part of your microbiome, named the Estrobolome, is made up of a collection of bacteria equipped with special genes that metabolize estrogen. When the estrobolome is not working optimally, women can experience abnormal estrogen levels resulting in irregular periods, disruptions in the menstrual cycle, impaired ovulation, polycystic ovary syndrome (PCOS), and endometriosis. All of these symptoms invariably point to infertility. Can you guess what can disturb the estrobolome? Again, chronic stress.

Let's say you're a woman, your hormonal HPA-HPG axes are in homeostasis, and you get pregnant. The composition of your maternal gut microbiome will contribute to outcomes with long-term health consequences for you and your child. To give you an idea of the centrality of the maternal gut flora, the genes contained within the human microbiota -- which produce metabolites, vitamins, enzymes, and hormones, to name a few -- are 150-fold greater than those contained within the individual human genome. That's a lot of intestinal territory and with the right — or rather wrong — environmental pressures, a lot can go haywire.

The job of the gut microbiome is as complex as that of cortisol, our hormone master. It assists us in the digestion of our own food components that we cannot handle, works along with the liver to detoxify and excrete injurious foreign chemicals, trains our immune system and defends us from invasion of dangerous pathogens. If the gut wall barrier - a one layer deep surface of epithelial cells covered by a thin layer of mucus, and intimately coexisting with the microbes nestled in there - is healthy, you'll be healthy. Without that healthy gut wall, however, there is trouble: the result is a "leaky gut," that is too permeable and no longer protects us from the external world. That epithelial layer of intestinal cells sits on top of the Gut Associated Lymphoid Tissue (GALT) where 70% of our immune system resides. If the other tasks weren't enough, the gut wall complex has the even more daunting task of protecting our bodies from potentially harmful microbes and toxins, while also allowing in nutrients and tolerating the commensal non-pathogenic microbes. Without a healthy intestinal wall, migrating pathogenic bacteria, toxins and chunks of protein from incompletely digested food end up in the circulation and lead to a host of conditions through chronic inflammation and immune activation. The consequences are more than a little annoying. Leaky gut can lead to diet-induced food sensitivities and is a known factor in celiac and Crohn's disease. Leaky gut has been associated with other autoimmune diseases[8] like lupus, type 1 diabetes, multiple sclerosis, chronic fatigue syndrome, fibromyalgia, arthritis, allergies, asthma, obesity, and even mental illness.

And so develops a perpetual vicious circle of stress, dysbiosis, gut inflammation and increased intestinal permeability.

Our microbiome is as unique to us as are our thumbprints. We can liken the gut microbiome to a vast city, with skyscrapers, streets, parks, vehicles, and people — all beautifully in sync with each other and doing its own job until some event perturbs this network of symbiotic relationships. Suddenly, this city, or rather, the gut microbiome, becomes vulnerable to negative environmental influences. One of these is birth by Cesarean section, typically the delivery method for babies in a breech, or tush-first, position leading up to labor. Research has shown that babies delivered by C-section do not come into contact with the mother's vaginal microbiome, and they do not "inherit" the microbes necessary to the important development of their own gut microbiome. Less clear is the relationship between the mother's gut microbiome and her breastfeeding status on the development of the infant's early gut microbiota.

The effect of stress on the microbiome is impressive - after only 2 hours of exposure to high salivary cortisol, the profiles of activities of the whole oral bacterial community had already changed and they were similar to the ones found in periodontitis progression, a serious and progressive gum infection.[9] Looks like a nice smile goes hand in hand with successful stress management.

We know, of course, that what we eat plays a significant role in determining the microbiome's functionality. Unfortunately, the Western diet, available to millions, perhaps billions, of us around the world is high in fat, sugar, and salt, and low in fiber and polyphenols that feed our good bacteria. So many of the processed foods we encounter in our bread, snack, and refrigerated supermarket aisles promote dysbiosis, an imbalance in our gut bacteria – as well as diminished microbial diversity. Indeed, transplanting the Western diet's dysbiotic microbiota into germ-free mice makes the mice fat.[10] It's frightening to consider that this loss of bacterial diversity has changed our gut microbiome over the past several decades. Moreover, high saturated fat diets, in particular, are known to induce inflammation in the gut and peripheral tissues. And inflammation promotes obesity.[11]

All is not hopeless! A high-fiber diet can help transform the type and amount of microbiota in the gut. Dietary fiber from prebiotic foods indeed feed specific bacteria strains in our microbiome, supporting production of short chain fatty acids (SCFA), such as acetate, propionate, and butyrate, that in turn "feed" other parts of the microbiome and the human gut wall cells of the colon. If you aren't already eating foods high in prebiotic fiber, such as garlic, onions, leeks, asparagus, Jerusalem artichokes, dandelion greens, bananas and seaweed, consider integrating them into several meals a week. Grass fed butter and ghee are good sources of butyrate.

The dietary fiber from these prebiotic foods is non-digestible in the small intestine, and fermentable by bacteria (broken down and fermented by microbiota enzymes in the colon). SCFA are released during the fermentation process. Consequently, the pH of the colon is reduced and encourages the growth of microbiota that will survive in this more acidic gut environment. Research has found that a lower pH value (less than "7") limits the growth of harmful bacteria such as *Clostridium difficile*. It's also shown that

SCFA stimulates immune cell activity and helps the body maintain normal blood levels of glucose and cholesterol.

A word of caution. If you've got a condition such as irritable bowel syndrome, you need to introduce prebiotics in small amounts so you can test your tolerance to them. There are numerous fiber types and different formulations of prebiotic fibers, and it is difficult to know which one is best for you. In the case of high-fiber foods, people who committed to a healthier lifestyle ultimately profit from a short-term unpleasant side effect: flatulence. The momentary discomfort has a payoff as a low-fiber diet reduces the amount of beneficial microbiota while also increasing the number of disease-inducing bacteria. It's best to consult with your doctor or dietician before making any dramatic change — even a good one — in your food consumption.

Another class of foods known as fermented foods can also ramp up your gut microbiome. They include yogurt, sauerkraut, kimchi, kombucha, pickles, miso, nattō and other fermented soybean and vegetable products. These foods, produced by bacterial fermentation, contain SCFA, which have a direct influence on metabolic functions. A 2021 study from Stanford University lead by Professor Justin Sonnenburg, and his group,[12] has studied the effect of a high plant-based fiber diet versus a high fermented food diet on the human gut microbiome. To his surprise, only the high-fermented-food diet steadily increased microbiota diversity, which is associated with good health, and decreased inflammatory markers. The conclusion: fermented foods may be valuable in countering the decreased microbiome diversity and increased inflammation pervasive with the Western diet.

Anecdotally speaking, we've all felt "sick to the stomach" when faced with depressing news. We've "lost our appetite" when we got upset. We've gotten "butterflies in our stomach" when we've been in uncomfortable situations or high emotional states. We "listen to our gut" to understand our feelings. Increasingly, researchers are addressing the bi-directional links between gut physiology and brain function, and they're explaining how these links operate under normal and stressful conditions. Most patients suffering from depression, anxiety, IBS and other functional brain-gut disorders are extremely sensitive to stressful events.

Germ free mice grow into adults that are hyper-responsive to stressful stimuli by producing corticosterone, equivalent to cortisol in humans. When researchers transplanted beneficial microbiota in their guts at an early age, these effects were reversed. Nevertheless the effect could not be achieved once the mice were adults. Traumatic life events, especially those acting on critical brain development window, serve as a prerequisite of the HPA axis dysregulation and aberrant immune-inflammatory processes. On the other side, abnormal solicitation of the HPA axis during the brain development can impact microbial colonization and visceral sensitivity, as it is suggested in irritable bowel syndrome.[13][14]

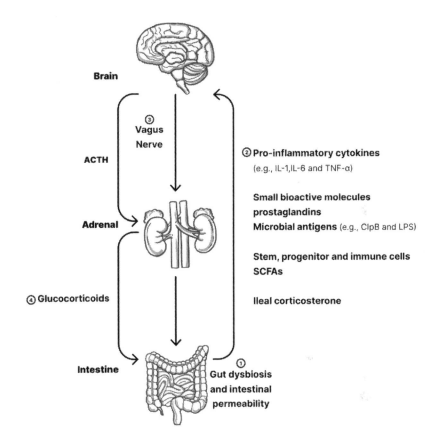

Fig. 1. Overview of mechanisms linking the gut microbiota and the HPA axis activity. The gut microbial alterations and increased intestinal permeability (1) lead to a release of various mediators, such as pro-inflammatory cytokines, microbial antigens and ileal corticosterone, as well as the mobilization of stem/progenitor cells that pass through the blood-brain barrier and activate the HPA axis (2). Short chain fatty acids (SCFAs) may attenuate the HPA axis.

Abbreviations: ACTH - adrenocorticotropic hormone; ClpB - caseinolytic peptidase B; IL-1 - interleukin-1, IL-6 - interleukin-6, LPS - lipopolysaccharide; SCFAs - short-chain fatty acids; TNF-α - tumor necrosis factor-α.

Adapted from : **The HPA axis dysregulation in severe**

mental illness: Can we shift the blame to gut microbiota?[15]

Optimally, gut-brain communication—modulated in part by cortisol and HPA Axis — ensures healthy coordination of gastrointestinal functions to support behavior and physiological processes. But a less than ideal external environment can upset the microbiome, which explains why we feel physically ill when we're under stress. In stress experiments, primarily done on laboratory animals, we learn that even short-term exposure to stress can impact the microbiota community profile by altering the relative proportions of gut bacteria. Indeed, researchers in a study called the Belgian Flemish Gut Flora Project[16] learned that *Coprococcus* and *Dialister*, two bacteria in the normal gut microbiome, are consistently depleted in depression. The project — one of the largest population-wide studies on the connection between gut flora and lifestyle — continues to examine the potential for microbial pathways to affect the brain and nervous system.

It's not your imagination: We can thank the gut-brain axis — and its cortisol "facilitator" — for the feeling of malaise or downright sickness that accompanies our feelings of depression.[17]

It's mind-blowing to think that microbes in your gut "talk" to your brain, thanks to the intervention of cortisol — and that they will shape your physical and mental destiny. Adhering to the old adage that there's strength in numbers, the gut microbiome — with as many as 400 trillion microbes — acts as another organ with the power to affect our health, behavior, and neurological life. Research on the gut-brain axis may not be as fast as we'd like: Studies are often ethically problematic and therefore tend to be performed on piglets, whose gut and brain development in infancy is remarkably similar to human infants. Through these animal studies, we're learning more and more about the relationships between bacteria in the gut and brain through metabolites — the intermediate or end products of cell metabolism. Some of these brain metabolites show up in altered states in people diagnosed with various disorders, such as autism.

In one study analysis, for example, researchers posited a possible three-way relationship between the gut bacteria *Ruminococcus*, the amino acid NAA, and cortisol. Using a statistical methodology, they discovered that *Ruminococcus* communicates with and makes changes to the brain directly through cortisol. This finding may give researchers insight into one way that the gut microbiota "talks" to the brain. It can be the basis for developing comparable studies of the gut-brain axis — and for bringing the goodness of gut microbiome research into our digestive, reproductive, social, and cognitive lives.

Takeaways

- The gut microbiome is critical to your health and wellbeing, and it is affected by stress and HPA dysregulation.

- Abnormal HPA axis reactivity, resulting in abnormal cortisol, changes the composition and activity of the gut microbiota.

- A normal cortisol is necessary for mucosal gut healing. Stress, dysbiosis, gut inflammation and increased intestinal permeability perpetuate each other in a vicious circle.

- There is a cross-talk between the HPA axis and the gut-brain axis.

Chapter 8

Cortisol and Weight Loss: Why So Many Diets Fail

We call the people we love "sweetie" and "honey." A horrid experience makes us feel sick to our stomach. We designate sweets and fats as "comfort food" and take refuge in binge eating them.

You don't have to know much about the gut-brain axis to recognize that food and mental outlook go together like burgers and fries, peanut butter and jelly — you get the message. The words we use in everyday conversation reveal the implicit connections we make with food, eating, and emotional outlook.

As with reproductive health, athletic fitness, peak metabolic functionality, and healthy mindset, eating — particularly the tendency to overeat and gain weight — is in large part shaped by cortisol. When you're feeling stress, or you're not getting eight hours of sleep at night, or if you're battling depression, the hypothalamic-pituitary-adrenal (HPA) axis gets activated and secretes corticotropin-releasing hormone (CRH) from the hypothalamus. CRH signals the anterior pituitary gland to release adrenocorticotropic hormone (ACTH). ACTH stimulates the release of cortisol from the adrenal gland, leading to a cascade of intricate physiological events. In a good scenario, when your stress diminishes, the cortisol response is terminated through a negative feedback loop: Cortisol suppresses further release of ACTH and CRH. In a scenario of ongoing stress, however, the feedback mechanism is impaired. Cortisol levels stay chronically high.

In stressful situations, many of us turn to food for comfort. Unfortunately, the emotions born of stress disrupt normal digestive functions — and maybe even your rational thinking. In more placid times, you're more likely to make healthy eating decisions. But elevated cortisol, incited by stress, more often than not, makes you reach for the carbs, sugar and salt. That's why we think of chips, pretzels, and chocolate bars as psychological comfort food when, in fact, they create discomfort in your gut — and your mind.

"Back in the day, science told us calories in, calories out," says author Shawn Talbott, who holds a Ph.D. in nutritional biochemistry. "But the science has evolved so that we began to see it's not strictly a math problem. It's essentially a problem of hormone and neurotransmitter signaling."[1]

Indeed, a 2016 Stanford University research study shows that in essence, the glucocorticoid stress hormones send a signal via a molecule called Adamts1 to make more fat cells. The study results do not exclude the possibility that other, as yet unknown, hormones also signal the fat cells to mature, but Adamts1 is likely one of the most important.[2]

Think about it, Talbott says. If losing weight were simply a matter of calories in, calories out, we wouldn't have a worldwide obesity crisis.

"Calories in, calories out is still important," Talbott says. "But the more we understand about the scientific thinking around appetite signaling, the more likely we are to eat better, maintain a healthy weight, sleep better, and feel better about our lives."

Despite the $33 billion that people in the US spend on weight-loss products a year, dieting is not the path to a healthy weight. In fact, dieting keeps your cortisol levels high. When it's activated by stress, cortisol keeps signaling your brain that you're hungry, especially for carbs. Once you've ingested those burgers, fries, doughnuts and chips, cortisol sends a potent signal to your belly fat cells to store as much fat as possible. Faster than you can say, "I'll have fries with that," you're carrying excess podge across your abdomen. That girth is the most dangerous kind of fat. It surrounds your internal organs and puts you at greater risk for developing heart disease, diabetes, liver problems and some types of cancer.

Hormones throughout the body are also engaged with the vagus nerve – the part of the parasympathetic nervous system that facilitates communication between the gastrointestinal tract and the brain. The relevant microbes in your gut microbiome release key transmitters designed to modulate food intake. These are primarily short-chain fatty acids, serotonin, hunger-initiating ghrelin and other biochemicals involved in digestion. When cortisol levels are normal, gut hormones signal the hypothalamus to say it's time to stop eating. When levels stay high, the brain doesn't get the memo. If you're eating processed food high in bad fat, sugar, emulsifiers, colorants and other chemicals, you're also perturbing the gut microbiome. You won't feel well. Your energy will flag. You'll still feel hungry and you'll keep eating.

We talked about the centrality of the gut microbiome and its responsiveness to cortisol — and it's also crucial to any discussion about obesity. To review briefly, something like 10^{14} microorganisms exist in the human gut microbiome, roughly a 1:1 ratio of bacteria to human cells.[3] Over the past couple of decades, researchers have learned that a healthy gut microbiota is able to stave off negative health conditions, such as type 2 diabetes, cardiovascular diseases, and obesity. These microbes — *Bacteroidetes* and *Firmicutes* make up 75% of them — are the frontline workers in the body that help the gut absorb, break down, and store nutrients. An imbalance in the gut microbiome stemming from a low-nutrient diet will promote the growth of organisms that cause chronic inflammation, chronic intestinal diseases and obesity.

Firmicutes, for example, frequently dominate the gut of obese individuals and help them extract more calories from the food they eat. By contrast, people who maintain a normal weight with a low-fat, high-fiber diet exhibit a decreased *Firmicutes* population.

Other microbes have been shown to help prevent obesity.

Studies indicate that *Bifidobacteria* — among the first microbes to colonize the human gastrointestinal tract — exert positive health benefits on the gut microbiome and, significantly, are less present in obese people. A recent study found that certain prebiotics, or compounds in food that induce the growth or activity of beneficial microorganisms, promote the growth of *Bifidobacteria*, which aid in stimulating signals along the vagus nerve to reduce fat.

We in the West face a real problem implementing what we've learned about the gut microbiome, because the food in our western diet has robbed the gut of "good bacteria." Indeed, the human gut throughout North America and Europe is largely characterized by reduced bacterial diversity and an increase in proinflammatory species that defines dysbiosis. Ironically, some westerners are inclined to associate Africa, for example, with underfed children. In reality, studies reveal that most African children who consume high fiber diets have greater diversity of intestinal microbes and fewer pathogenic, or disease-inducing, bacteria.[4] These children also possess larger amounts of healthful *Bacteroidetes* than European children. The western diet rich in sugar, fats, chemicals and poor in fiber and fermented foods reduces intestinal microbial diversity. Whereas most people had balanced cortisol and insulin levels a century ago, we see now that current-day people in the West have been starving their gut microbiome of the nourishment it needs to avoid obesity, inflammation, and a host of cognitive issues, including Alzheimer's Disease.

Our western diet is also responsible for pasteurized and germ-free foods that tend to decrease the gut's satiety peptides — the short chains of amino acids that reduce appetite and limit our desire for more and more food. Our continuous ingestion of processed foods, stripped clean of fiber, pasteurized, chemically preserved with unpronounceable additives to extend supermarket shelf life and emulsifiers that strip the mucus layer, and flavored with sugar, salt, and fat, does not promote gut health and metabolic flexibility. Obese individuals secrete fewer of these satiety peptides. The consequence of excess body fat, especially around the belly, and lack of exercise is insulin resistance. That's when the insulin receptors in your cells refuse to open up for sugar to be used. Your glucose has difficulty getting out of your bloodstream and cannot be easily used for energy. To compensate, the pancreas starts to make more insulin. The body's workaround isn't very efficient though, because your blood sugar levels just keep going up. Many individuals with these biochemical events are eventually diagnosed with hyperglycemia. The body cries, "It's just too hard to get out of this vicious cycle!"

Figure 2

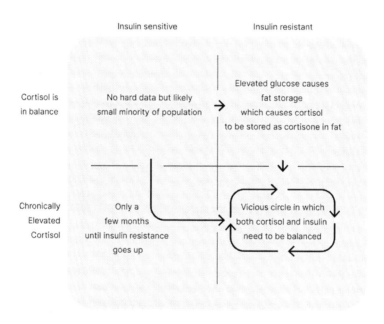

A quadrant relationship between cortisol and insulin

Overweight, insulin resistance, and type 2 diabetes all get stuck in a vicious circle with cortisol.[56] The result is often metabolic syndrome, with increases in blood pressure, elevated blood sugar, intra-abdominal fat deposits, elevated serum triglycerides, and risk for heart attack and stroke.

Some food researchers encourage us to fast to reproduce the conditions under which our metabolism decreases our body's sugar levels and increases its capacity to burn surplus fat.

"Intermittent fasting tends to raise cortisol, " says nephrologist and author Jason Fung, MD. "That's normal! Cortisol is in sync with your circadian rhythm. It's high in the morning and subsides as the day goes along. If you're doing intermittent fasting, you won't constantly get those highs of insulin from your food."[7]

Let's take a look at the various fasting stages in Figure 3. Column #1 shows the various stages of processes in your body after you stop eating food. (You should continue to drink calorie-free fluids.) Column #2 shows the number of hours post-food intake. Column #3 shows the effects on your body areas measured by the level of ketones in your blood.[8] Ketones are substances the body makes from your fat when your glucose supply gets low.

Figure 3
The stages in intermittent fasting

Fasting Stages	Hours elapsed post-eating	Effects
Stage 1	8+	Stable Blood Sugar
Stage 2	24+	Ketosis,* Fat Burning, and Mental Clarity
Stage 3	36-72+	Autophagy and Anti-Aging? **

Ketosis is a state when the body doesn't have enough carbohydrates to burn for energy and switches to burning fat producing ketones. This means that the glucose stored in the liver and muscles (glycogen) will be used up first before the body turns to ketones.

** *See* https://www.sciencedirect.com/science/article/pii/ S1568163718301478 and https://www.nature.com/articles/ nmeth.3661.

Of particular note is the process of autophagy, which means eating oneself. After 36-72 hours of fasting, our body goes into a cleaning mode where it recycles misfolded proteins, defective cell parts, and pro-inflammatory "zombie cells." Autophagy will rejuvenate the immune system, grow stem cells, and may prevent cancer. Further research is sure to reveal additional benefits of autophagy.[9]

When you fast by extending the period during which your body burns through the calories you consumed in your last meal, you follow a? time-restricted eating?. That is great news for your body, which gets a rest for housekeeping functions and realigns itself with the circadian rhythm. Fasting is not as distasteful as it sounds, because you're not starving yourself. You're simply delimiting the hours in which you're going to eat. There are several versions of time-restricted eating, you'll confine yourself to eating three times a day without snacking, at 8:00 AM., noon, and 6:00 PM, or eat once a day at 7:00 PM for example.? The goal is to give your body time to start to burn fat and reprogram your eating habits, so they are intentional and life-sustaining.

We're of the mind that an eating schedule makes the most sense. There are numerous books on fasting. If you're going to go in any extreme direction — say, eating only one meal a day, two days each week — we'd want you first to consult with your doctor or nutritionist. If you're in an unrelentingly high-stress situation, even healthier eating habits won't bring your cortisol levels down. In this case, it's time to seek counseling help and follow the recommendations at the end of this book. Don't forget: Your cortisol measurements give you an incremental picture of what's going on inside you at the biochemical, emotional, and psychological levels. No other biomarker can reliably offer you this actionable detail.

In the US, 73.6 percent of American adults — 190 million people — are overweight or obese (BMI 25+).[10] In the EU, some 52.7 percent of the adult population is overweight.[11] Food researchers say that women and men in both population sets have become equally obese because of excessive secretion of cortisol, along with reduced secretion of key anabolic hormones necessary for metabolism, including dehydroepiandrosterone (DHEA), testosterone, and growth hormone. This combination of reduced anabolic hormones and highly catabolic cortisol makes the body lose muscle, slow metabolic rate, increase appetite, and store fat, primarily in the abdomen. Stress makes all of us, women and men, burn fewer calories and eat more, especially carbs, which further exacerbates our stress levels. The vicious cycle again!

The belief persists, nevertheless, that more women than men are obese. Indeed, Harvard Medical School (HMS) has published work suggesting that women and men have different "stress-coping behavior," with women turning to food for comfort and men choosing alcohol or cigarettes. Moreover, HMS writes, a Finnish study of more than 5,000 men and women showed that obesity was associated with stress-related eating in women but not in men.

Let's see what additional research says.

One Yale University study looked at two groups of young women. Half of the women had a high level of "cognitive dietary restraint;" that is, they consciously refrained from eating certain foods. The other half was less focused on dieting. Yet, the first group that restricted its food intake had significantly higher cortisol levels – while also getting more exercise.[12] The Yale scientists showed that high levels of stress, in fact, increase cortisol levels. Moreover, they went on to link high cortisol levels to accumulation of abdominal body fat in both men and women, even in healthy, young, lean people.

A group of Italian researchers investigated the dynamics of weight gain in obese adult pre-menopausal women after a "well-defined stressful event," and compared this group to other obese women not experiencing stress.[13] The study found that the stressed-out obese women gained weight rapidly after an important stressful event and exhibited "overactivated adrenocortical function," which persisted over time even after the stressful event ended. The researchers observed too that glucocorticoids had a "direct impact" on the ability of adipose, or fatty, tissue to burn fat, and that they "downregulated," or suppressed, lipase - an enzyme that breaks down fats in food so they can be absorbed in the intestine. Glucocorticoids also suppressed thermogenesis, the body's mechanism to produce the heat necessary for burning calories; interfered with leptin, a hormone that helps the body maintain a normal weight on a long-term basis; and increased visceral adiposity – fat accumulating in the abdomen surrounding body organs. As with all events that perturb the HPA, glucocorticoids increase the expression of cortisol releasing factor (CRF) mRNA, which "locks in" the stress response, and along with insulin, stimulates the desire for your favorite unhealthy comfort foods.

More bad news: Chronically *stressed* obese women, who diet and lose weight, are candidates for relapse: Once they've lost weight, they start overeating again.

Richard J. Johnson, professor of renal diseases and hypertension at the University of Colorado-Denver, has located this phenomenon in a mechanism he terms the "fat switch," whereby animal physiology "flips" an ancient "switch," triggered through fructose and uric acid, that once ensured weight gain during times of food scarcity. Despite living in times of plenty, modern-day women have retained this evolutionary fat switch – and we eat as if there's no tomorrow. Just as in more aboriginal times, our food is converted into fat and stored in our body:[14] We treat every meal as if it's our last.

When we overeat, the body's visceral fat cells – fat stored deep inside the belly and wrapped around the organs – expand and cortisol gets stored as cortisone. The fat cells become cortisol-releasing glands. When you least need it, cortisol "comes out of hiding" and increases your glucose levels. And every time you eat, your cortisol goes up. Even at a healthy weight, chronic stress packs on the pounds and insulin resistance takes hold. Diet and stress researchers have known for decades that stress leads to emotional eating – which, in turn, increases stress, cortisol, and craving for comfort food.[15]

What about men?

A US-Swedish team of researchers recruited 1,302 men from Sweden's National Population Register to study the impact of stress on their cortisol levels, body mass index (BMI), testosterone levels, blood pressure, and other bodily factors. Looking at cortisol levels throughout the day via salivary measurements, the researchers found that the male subjects had an activated HPA axis and inhibited HPG and growth hormone (GH) axes. In other words, stress-related cortisol secretion showed negative effects on testosterone, insulin-like growth factor 1 (IGF-1), and high density lipids (HDL), popularly known as the "good cholesterol." Obese men were prone to lower sex steroid and GH activity and they suffered from fatty tissue in various areas of the body, notably the abdomen. The men experienced these endocrine reactions as feelings of defeat and helplessness.

When it comes to the harmful effects on obese individuals, cortisol is an equal opportunity employer. The main difference lies in testosterone and estrogen/progesterone levels: An obese woman with a "stressed out" HPG axis will likely have trouble getting pregnant, and an obese man with the same HPG axis profile will have trouble producing enough testosterone to maintain his normal sexual development and functionality. He would almost certainly be dealing with a cluster of other health-related problems involving insulin and glucose levels, cholesterol, high blood pressure, LDL-cholesterol, or the "bad cholesterol."

Stress eating doesn't happen overnight. Sadly, it often starts in childhood and knows no geographical boundaries. North and South America can claim 75 million obese children. The Western Pacific Region: 84 million; Southeast Asia: 47 million; Eastern Mediterranean: 42 million; Africa: 43 million; and Europe: 41 million. Without intervention, obese children grow into obese adults with hypertension and metabolic disorders. They have lower self-esteem than children in a normal weight range. Their school attendance levels are poor and their academic achievements are frequently low. Their prospects for well-paying, meaningful work are lower than for more physically fit children.[16] It's no wonder that Liesbeth van Rossum, an internist-endocrinologist and co-founder of the Obesity Center (Centrum Gezond Gewicht) at the Erasmus Medical Center in Rotterdam, calls obesity a "gateway disease to many other diseases," and believes cortisol should be a biomarker for weight loss second only to insulin.

It's safe to assume that in women, men, and children, chronically high cortisol levels turn on the cortisol fat switch, in which excessive cortisol gets stored in visceral fat as cortisone, and then re-activated, leading to further weight gain. Even when obese individuals successfully avoid stressful situations, their normal cortisol levels are at the mercy of an enzyme inside fat cells called 11β-Hydroxysteroid dehydrogenase type 1 (HSD-1): When cortisol has done its job and has become deactivated, HSD type 1 can reactivate cortisone from the fat cells and turn it into cortisol. And the whole confounding food craving cycle starts all over again.

German researchers, among others, are studying the genetic basis for the HSD-1 enzyme and its correlation with chronic stress, restrained eating (dieting), and sleep deprivation. Already they have learned that foods rich in flavonoids, such as apples, onions, grapefruit, soybeans, coffee, and especially oranges, help control HSD's sabotaging behavior.[17] Black licorice contains a flavonoid called glycyrrhetinic acid that inhibits HSD, but has to be used sparingly, because it also raises blood pressure.

We didn't write *this book* to bring you to despair. By measuring your cortisol levels, we know you can — and will — get a handle on your brain response through this mysterious, shape-shifting stress hormone.

Takeaways

- It's physiologically impossible to lose weight long term when cortisol is out of balance - through the cortisol fat switch, fat gets stored in the worst place, inside your abdomen around your organs.

- Stress makes us burn fewer calories and eat more (especially carbs).

- The "fat switch" – a fat-storage mechanism reaching back to the earliest days of our species – may be the #1 cause of difficulty losing weight.

- Intermittent fasting gives your body time to become metabolically flexible, and switch from burning sugar to burning fat.

Chapter 9

Cortisol for The Diagnosis of Long Covid?

Elevated cortisol secretion is considered to be a central part in a well-orchestrated immune response to stress, including illness. Cortisol has an essential role in immune cell trafficking, by directing migration of lymphocytes, monocytes and eosinophil immune cells into affected body compartments or sites of inflammation. These effects help reduce the risk for infections.[1] Another major attribute of cortisol-stress response is that it restrains the excessive inflammatory reaction.

The recently unveiled National Research Plan on Long COVID[2] on August 3rd of this year, acknowledges that research is urgently needed to understand the biological mechanisms that underpin the more than 200 symptoms and signs and 50 conditions attributed to Long COVID and to develop evidence-based treatments for them.

Long COVID[3] is defined as "a multifaceted disease that can affect nearly every organ system" and can manifest as new or worsening chronic health problems, including but not limited to heart disease, diabetes, kidney disease, hematologic issues, and mental and neurologic conditions. The signs, symptoms, and conditions continue or start 4 weeks or more after the initial symptomatic or asymptomatic infection and may be relapsing and remitting.

"Long Covid needs to be elevated to a national priority on par with vaccines and antiviral therapeutics," argues a group of 53 scientists in their Covid-19 strategic roadmap,[4] spearheaded by Ezekiel Emanuel, MD, co-director of the Healthcare Transformation Institute at the University of Pennsylvania.

About twenty percent[5] – more than half in other studies[6] – of patients report Long Covid with symptoms like chronic fatigue, shortness of breath, sleep abnormalities, headache, brain fog, joint pains, nausea, cough, and abdominal pain.[7] This means tens of millions of people are affected, and in the U.S. alone, 4 million are out of work because of Long Covid, 2.4% of the working population.[8]

Earlier scientific papers have linked cortisol with Long Covid: Long Covid symptoms can be explained by low cortisol due to a SARS-CoV2 action on adrenal glands.[9,10] Depression and fatigue are positively correlated with cortisol in Long Covid.[11]

In an article published in Nature in May 2022, the authors opined that adrenal gland insufficiency in patients with COVID-19 might be induced through different mechanisms, including vascular damage, viral replication, inflammatory factors and improper tapering off of long-term steroid replacement.[12]

On August 10, 2022, a breakthrough Yale University study,[13] promptly covered by mass media,[14,15,16] was pre-published by Jon Klein et al. The Yale immunology lab, led by Professor Akiko Iwasaki, has been at the forefront of Covid research. And even though there are the necessary caveats – it has to go through peer review and should not be used to guide clinical practice (yet) – this new study builds on the cortisol papers referenced above.

In 2004, after the SARS outbreak in Hong Kong, scientists already noticed the effect of the virus on the HPA Axis and cortisol.[17] Autopsies revealed that cortisol-producing cells in the adrenal gland showed degeneration and necrosis.[18] In fact, SARS (the first infamous Covid strain) showed as well that the body breaks down the cortisol response by itself.[19] Our bodies produce antibodies to counter the virus, but they look like our own hormone ACTH. So instead of attacking the virus, we're binding our own antibodies with ACTH, which happens to be the hormone initiating cortisol secretion . This is one possible explanation why cortisol levels drop in Long Covid. SARS CoV9 virus is also capable of infecting the adrenal cells (which express ACE-

2 receptors), and replicating intracellularly, leading to cell death by several mechanisms.

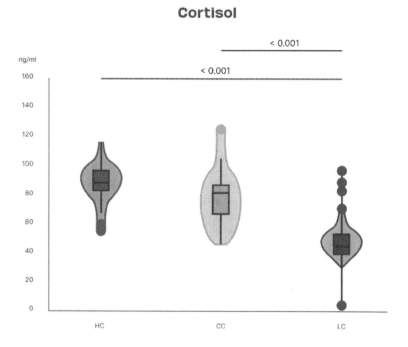

As you can see in the graph from the Yale study,[20] Long Covid (LC) shows a 50% decrease in serum morning cortisol levels vs. normal cortisol levels (HC) in? recovered patients (CC).? The symptoms of Long Covid overlap with those of Hypocortisolism. Cortisol clearly distinguishes those who developed Long Covid from normal and recovered subjects.

Further studies are needed to prove whether cortisol, and which of cortisol's parameters, **could be used as diagnosis for Long Covid**.[21]

Salivary cortisol determination has been recommended in some studies for establishing and monitoring Long Covid recovery plans.[22] While this represents great progress, more studies are needed to validate these learnings, including the precise role of salivary cortisol testing at home, in the diagnosis and management of Long Covid.

Hopefully, cortisol saliva tests will be validated for Long Covid and allow consumers to test their cortisol levels at home within minutes without the need for a lab. Until more data are available, we cannot make any strong statements here. There is currently no widely adopted standard for measuring Long Covid, and any claim that home cortisol testing would be a diagnostic tool, or is beneficial in the recovery, would be counterproductive at this point in time. Any health decision should be made after consulting your physician.

We've written before about how cortisol increases the risk of catching Covid.[23] Several scientific papers have been published about cortisol and Covid in 2020 and 2021:

- High Cortisol increases the risk of attracting Covid.[24]

- High Cortisol increases mortality after attracting Covid.[25][26][27]

- Cortisol is an independent predictor of unfavorable outcomes in hospitalized Covid patients.[28]

Chapter 10

Scientific Breakthrough: Mindset Controls Cortisol

Are you as awestruck by Shadrack's athletic prowess as we are? It's incredible that the mindset Shadrack brought to his running life in the face of a potentially career-ending injury could help determine his cortisol levels. We had to ask: Can an affirmative outlook like his also balance cortisol levels in a stressful non-athletic context? We didn't expect the answer to lie simply in adopting one relaxation technique over another. There are hundreds of mindfulness, mind-over-matter, behavioral, and positive-thinking methodologies on the market, each one touting its effectiveness, yet Shadrack hadn't used any of them. He had acquired a holistic approach to his stress: He saw himself as a whole person, not just an athlete, not just a student, not just a patient. Could a strong mindset — whatever that may be — in fact help the body produce cortisol that responds dynamically to stress, increasing or decreasing hormonal secretion as needed?

What Shadrack and other talented athletes have learned through dogged personal experience has long attracted the attention of behavioral researchers, beginning with endocrinologist Hans Selye, who described stress as the "nonspecific response of the body to any demand," and who was the first scientist to link the HPA axis to the body's biological response to stress. Among more recent researchers is Alia Crum. We've cited Professor Crum throughout our book because her research at the Stanford Mind & Body Lab on mindsets is powerfully relevant to our own exploration of stress and cortisol. That's why we're devoting an entire chapter to her work. Her observations about mindsets, we

SCIENTIFIC BREAKTHROUGH: MINDSET CONTROLS CORTISOL

believe, will help you keep your cortisol levels in homeostatic balance.

Unlike so many researchers and pop culture pundits who view stress as a public health nemesis, Crum and her colleagues posit that the "stress mindset is a distinct variable that influences the stress response," a factor just as discrete as amount and severity of stress. Moreover, Crum says, an individual's attitude can either prolong or shorten stress. She talks about a "stress-is-enhancing" mindset to describe the belief that stress has "enhancing consequences for various stress-related outcomes, such as performance and productivity, health and well-being, and learning and growth," as opposed to a "stress-is-debilitating" mindset, whereby people believe stress has debilitating outcomes, such as depression and poor health. In her seminal work,[1] she and her co-authors write that from an evolutionary standpoint, the stress response, originating in the HPA axis, improves physiological and mental functioning "to meet imminent demands and enable survival."

In short, stress is a complex biological and psychological phenomenon intended to let us assess our environment to make sure we're safe.

Implied in Crum's analysis: We are equipped by nature to handle stress whatever its source, be it a saber-toothed tiger or a college entrance exam. In these cases or any other, we learn to marshal our inner resources to survive physical danger or mental anxiety.[2]

"Our work at the Mind & Body Lab has tried to get people (a) to realize that the negative effects of stress are only one side of the coin and we need to be aware of the positive effects of the stress response, and (b) to realize that our mindsets about stress help shape the stress response." Crum told us.

Crum's work reaches into the everyday activities of our lives. One study, for example, in which she and her colleagues measured salivary cortisol levels, students were asked by a Stanford Business School lecturer to prepare a speech about charisma. The students had ten minutes to write and would be selected at random to give the speech to a class of 100. The classmates would rate each speaker on their charisma.

"We found that most people tend to take on one of two profiles," Crum says. "Some people freaked out. In these cases, we saw highly elevated cortisol compared to their baseline. Their bodies and minds were engaged, but over-activated."

Crum says the other group of students were at the opposite extreme. They had mentally and emotionally checked out. "Their cortisol levels didn't move much from their baseline," she says. "If anything, their levels had even dropped."

The results of the study were not all that mystifying to Crum. "We've all seen these two types of people," she says. "Some take a task super-seriously and freak out. Some decide right from the start that they don't want to deal with the challenge and they retreat into themselves. The people in the latter group sort of hope they don't get picked. Neither freaking out, nor checking out, is a particularly adaptive response — and our cortisol measurements confirmed that."

Crum also recognized a small group of students who were engaged and physiologically aroused to an appropriate degree. They were able to focus on the task, view it as a surmountable challenge, and prepare to do their best in the event they were chosen to speak. Their cortisol levels were in the desired middle range of cortisol response, occupying a golden mean, or middle way, between two extremes.

To some degree, Crum's work with mindsets dovetails with comparable work she has done with the placebo effect — the sense of relative well-being that stems from unwittingly taking a sugar pill or engaging in a sham procedure because you believe the intervention is therapeutic.

"Your mindset is a major factor driving the placebo effect," Crum says. "In some studies, participants actually receive an

SCIENTIFIC BREAKTHROUGH: MINDSET CONTROLS CORTISOL

'honest placebo.' They're told that the intervention is a placebo — and research shows that the honest placebo also has positive effects. So, mindset is one mechanism through which the placebo effect works. At the Mind & Body Lab, we believe that promoting mindsets is a lot less deceptive, and more 'self-actualizing,' than kind of manipulating people through sugar pills."

In the course of her decades-long research, Crum wondered if people reacted to healthy food the way her student test participants had reacted to preparing a speech on charisma. Did they approach eating a healthy diet with a sense of purpose — even pleasure — or did they dread nutritious food as a necessary evil best avoided?

Almost anyone living in the western world will attest that foods typically found in the interior of supermarkets — snacks, sugary drinks, and foods with long lists of ingredients we can't pronounce — are, well, food in name only. The sugar and high fructose corn syrup added to these packaged, highly processed products have contributed to a genuine public health crisis, with some 422 million[3] people worldwide living with diabetes.[4] The disease occurs when your blood glucose, or blood sugar, is too high. You can largely avoid diabetes by "shopping the perimeter" at the supermarket, as food author Michael Pollan says, where you'll find vegetables, fish, lean meat, eggs and dairy.

We sympathize with you, though, if you have a hard time saying "no" to the salty, sugary, and fatty snacks that constitute two-thirds of the typical American supermarket. These goods are designed to be addictive so that "nobody can just eat one," as an old ad jingle used to boast. In the world most of us know, eating healthy foods often demands Herculean self-control.

Or does it?

As a graduate student at Yale, Crum worked with two professors — Kelly Brownell and Peter Salovey — "to test whether physiological satiation as measured by the gut peptide, ghrelin, may vary depending on the mindset in which one approaches consumption of food." In layman's terms, Crum was asking, "Do our beliefs about what we're eating change the body's physiological response to that food?"

She and her colleagues crafted a seemingly simple experiment. Study participants came into the lab thinking they were testing two different kinds of milkshakes. In Week #1, they were consuming a high-fat, caloric, indulgent-labeled milkshake. In Week #2, the same participants were told they were consuming a low-fat, low-calorie, sensible-labeled shake. The kicker: Both milkshakes were exactly the same. In this study, Crum et al were measuring ghrelin, the so-called "hunger hormone." A rise in ghrelin signals the brain to want more food. A drop in ghrelin tells the brain, "You don't need to eat so much any more." It revs up the metabolism to burn the nutrients you just ingested.

When Crum and her colleagues compared the consumption of the two milkshakes, they saw a threefold drop in ghrelin levels when participants thought they were consuming the high-fat, high-caloric, indulgent milkshake. Essentially, their bodies responded as if they had consumed more food and were fully satiated, even though they had consumed exactly the same milkshake in weeks #1 and #2.

"I think this was one of the first studies to show that your mindset — your preconceived notion about what you're eating — can physiologically decide how your body is going to respond to the food you eat," Crum says. "I had gone in thinking the better mindset to be in when you eat is that you're eating healthy. Ha! The results show the exact opposite. When our participants thought they were eating sensibly, their bodies left them feeling physiologically hungry. It seems if you want to lose or maintain weight, what's the best mindset to have? That you're eating indulgently! The ghrelin pathway is susceptible to thoughts!"

SCIENTIFIC BREAKTHROUGH: MINDSET CONTROLS CORTISOL

Ah, so that's why diets fail us! As Crum learned, your diet matters, but so does what you think about your diet. And so does what everyone around you thinks about your diet. Social contexts inform our mindsets. And our mindsets can change our physiology.

"But let's not get dualistic and say, 'It's all in the mind or it's not in the mind,'" Crum says. "And let's not be unnecessarily combative and say, 'Oh, my diet should be all plant-based, or keto, or whatever.' In some cases, if you think you should be adhering to a specific diet, and you're not, you'd actually be adding more stress to your life!"

Crum brilliantly demonstrated the mindset effect in 2007 when she and Harvard psychologist, Ellen Langer, asked 84 hotel housekeepers, working in seven different hotels, if they thought they were getting enough exercise. The average response was something like 3 on a scale of 1-10, with "10" indicating "I get a lot more exercise than most people." A third said they were getting zero exercise. Indeed, they had a mindset that positioned hotel work as work, not exercise.

Crum and Langer told half of the hotel workers that the work they do to clean hotel rooms was good exercise and satisfied the US Surgeon General's recommendations for an active lifestyle. The other half, the control group, was told nothing. Four weeks after the intervention, the informed group now believed they were getting sufficient exercise. In comparison with the control group, the informed group showed astonishing results: They showed a decrease in weight, blood pressure, body fat, waist-to-hip ratio, and body mass index. And yet, objectively speaking, nothing had changed. The hotel workers — all women — hadn't added yoga or push-ups to their daily routine. You can't make this stuff up: These results supported Crum and Langer's hypothesis: The mindset you bring to an activity plays a significant role in shaping your body's biochemistry.[5]

Best of all, the hotel housekeepers began feeling better about themselves, their bodies, and their work.

You've noticed, of course, that Crum's charisma speech study measured her participants' cortisol levels, but neither her milkshake study, nor her hotel worker exercise study, used cortisol as a biometric. We asked Professor Crum pointblank: Would knowing your participants' cortisol levels, in any future work you do around stress, anxiety, fear, or burnout, be useful to you — and to your participants?

Crum responds, ""We train people to become aware of their mindset. By measuring cortisol, we start to be aware of what is physiologically happening with our bodies. You have influence over how your body responds in part by changing your mindset. If mindsets are as powerful as we've seen them to be, it stands to reason that cortisol — like ghrelin — is something you control. You can tap into it through conscious and autonomic processes. That's empowering."

As Professor Crum concludes, your cortisol levels can shape your response to stress, and your mind can manage cortisol's behavior. "It's all kind of bidirectional, right?" she says. "But for me the question remains, how do you get a handle on your cortisol?"

If anyone can begin to answer this question, it's Alia Crum.[6] In the meantime, we want to tell you we've got your back. Once you measure your cortisol and understand what the numbers mean, we assert that whatever approach you take — whether it's believing in a higher power, adding yoga to your exercise routine, showing a commitment to self-care, turning up at a therapist's office every week, or realizing that it's time to rethink the way you handle stress — we want you to absorb your practice or ideas into every part of your life. As Shadrack Kipchirchir has. As Alia Crum has. We ourselves take our inspiration from them and so many others who are now looking at this "overlooked piece of the puzzle." Undoubtedly, looking stress in the eye — looking at

SCIENTIFIC BREAKTHROUGH: MINDSET CONTROLS CORTISOL

your cortisol numbers head on — can be sobering. But just ask yourself: Am I the same person at the end of this book as I was at the beginning?

You're already a different person.

So are we.

Like you, we've tried everything to manage our emotions, or our eating, or our couch potato habits. But because the world didn't know how important cortisol was, all our best efforts didn't get us to where we wanted to go. Now that we know what a critical role cortisol plays in our emotional, psychological and physical lives, we're better equipped to take great strides forward.

Let's keep going. You've already taken that first important step. We're with you. We're ready to embark on a better life with a mindset that works for, not against, us.

Takeaways

- You can manage your cortisol's behavior with a healthy mindset.

- Approaching your diet with an optimistic, "indulgent" mindset will help you manage your weight.

- You can tap into a good mindset through training, based on a solid scientific foundation.

Chapter 11

Recommendations: How to Keep Your Cortisol Levels Balanced

You want to lose weight.
    You want to rebound from some emotionally tough times.
    You want to get pregnant.
    You want to become your "personal best" athlete.
    Becoming who you want to become isn't going to be easy. But we're building a mobile home testing and recommendation engine on Pardigm.com, the first company in the world to do so, to assist you, beginning in 2023. We're going to do this both by helping you understand why it's so important that you measure your HPA axis stress response through cortisol levels, and then how these measurements can restore you to good mental health, prime physical form, and reproductive fertility.
    The recommendations you'll find here apply to most of the cortisol curve categories you encountered in Chapter 2: "Why You Should Measure Your Cortisol Levels." We're also including two more topics that we found intriguing. One is about hormetic stress, or using mild stressors to make your body and mind more robust. The other is if you should or not be skipping breakfast – practically a sacrilege in a country that has touted the notion for a century that breakfast is the most important meal of the day. You may very well be surprised where you come down on these two controversial subjects.

Unless you're holed up in a Zen monastery on the top of the Himalayas, you're going to be affected by chronic stress at some

RECOMMENDATIONS: HOW TO KEEP YOUR CORTISOL LEVELS BA...

point in your life. Looking around, we think it might be now. The good news is that cortisol imbalances, brought about by chronic stress, are responsive to lifestyle changes. You won't see improvement overnight, but if you're patient, and you're committed, you'll be able to reestablish the "circadian rhythmicity" and normalize your high or low levels of cortisol. As Dr. Sarah Berga told us, hormones speak in patterns, not just levels, and people feel the patterns more.

"Levels were only a small piece of the puzzle, and the pattern of pulses was the vast majority of it," she says. "The question we needed to answer was, 'What turns the pattern off?'"

To restore cortisol balance, you'll want to re-orchestrate the interactions of hormones in the HPA axis, other imbalanced hormones and neurotransmitters .

To accomplish this goal, you'll act at several levels:

1) **Control the stressors** you can modify: perceived stress, circadian rhythm/sleep alignment, blood sugar control, chronic inflammation, nutrition, and exercise

2) **Support your HPA axis** (brain and adrenal glands) and tweek the cortisol receptors and cortisol metabolism (11betaHSD1)

3) **Increase resilience to stress - mind and body**

How can you possibly do this? Let's dive into it.

1) Control the stressors

As Alia Crum at the Stanford Mind and Body Lab has told us, "Your mindset toward stress informs how your body reacts to it."

As we just mentioned , the first level is to address modifiable stressors:

Perceived stress

Perceived stress can be measured - see Perceived Stress Scale. [1] You might be amused to hear that it is characterized by N.U.T.S. factors: Novelty, Unpredictability, Threat to physiological or physiological well being, and Sense of loss of control.

Your mind must continuously send your body messages that it is safe, well nourished, supported, and calm in order for healing to occur and cortisol patterns to be optimal. Our brains are wired to detect threats through our eyes, nose, ears, and other senses, then analyze them through the brain's limbic system (amygdala, hippocampus and hypothalamus belong to it). By comparing the potential threat with past similar events, a decision is made to initiate (or not) the stress response, involving both Autonomic Nervous System (sympathetic and parasympathetic) and HPA Axis. That's why, for example, a certain smell can evoke a strong emotional and sometimes painful response. In humans, the limbic system is under the influence of the prefrontal cortex, our higher power and executive function brain area, capable of consciously overriding the perceived stressor. That is, unless our cortisol is chronically high, when the communication gets blurry.

I am refreshing your memory so you can understand the plethora of practices, apps, and devices that plug in at each step: mind-body interventions like yoga, meditation, echo meditation, emotional freedom technique, self-hypnosis, biofeedback, and tai-chi; autonomic system and parasympathetic/vagus nerve practices and devices; limbic system retraining; journaling, coloring and hobbies; your senses; body work, ... the list goes on and grows by the day. You have options, some better studied than others. Start with Chapter 10.

You can try to dampen the effect of the stressors by relying on your senses. While its effectiveness and mechanism are unclear, aromatherapy can help reduce stress. Researchers at the

School of Nursing at Youngnam Foreign Language College in Korea, for example, found that aroma inhalation could be an effective stress management method for high school students.[2]

Indeed, the olfactory nerve sends signals almost instantaneously to many parts of the brain, including the limbic system and amygdala, which are in charge of emotions, mood, and memory. These systems are also in charge of regulating our autonomic nervous system, which can either trigger a fight-or-flight response, or soothe us through turning on the parasympathetic nervous system to relax our bodies. This cascade of biophysical events helps explain why scents trigger our physical reactions and have lasting effects even years after the scent is gone.

Lavender, for example, has been shown to interact the same way biochemically that many anti-anxiety medications do on neuroreceptors. Lemon or yuzu, an east Asian citrus fruit, bergamot, clary sage, jasmine, and ylang ylang, a southeast Asian essential oil, have also aided in tamping down stress in various tense situations.

Spending time in nature too, has been found to lower blood pressure, heart rate, and levels of harmful hormones, including cortisol. The Japanese call this time spent in a natural setting *shin-rin-yoku*, or "nature-bathing." No actual bathing is required: Just a willingness to walk on a forest trail, find a bench or log where you can experience the sensation of the breeze on your skin, or inhale the scent of forest or ocean.

You might have not been aware of other common factors that our body perceives as stressful and we can modify:

Circadian rhythm alignment

How often are we told that a good night's sleep is the road to good health? That's all well and good. But why is sleep so important?

Your HPA axis and body's circadian rhythm reinforce each other and cortisol plays a major role. The CAR is an expression of it. Here, timing is essential, because we can reprogram the HPA axis by manipulating the three strongest signals: dark/light cycle with sleep, timing of food availability – time restricted eating – and the time when we move – move throughout the day, exercise in AM.

Sleep

Sleep is a crucial element of HPA axis recovery and cortisol balancing. And for the more severe cases, non-negotiable. Please sleep eight hours or more and, when you can, wake up without an alarm.

The body needs the right amount and pattern of cortisol to manage our circadian rhythm, or sleep-wake cycle.

Studies show that people with chronic sleep problems, such as apnea and insomnia, have higher cortisol levels during the day. Your body may be stimulating more alertness to counteract your lack of rest.

On the other hand, if you often find yourself wide awake in the middle of the night, please check your cortisol right then. High cortisol levels can also disrupt your sleep, causing further insomnia and fatigue. You've got to interrupt this unhealthy cycle.

Do what you do with small children:
Create a bedroom routine and stick to it every evening.
Here are some pointers:
Go to bed well before midnight. Aim for 10 PM.
Use your Fitbit, Oura or any other good fitness device or app, to measure the quality of sleep.
If you can't sleep through the night, consult with a sleep specialist (usually a pulmonologist). You may have to do a sleep

test to see if you have sleep apnea, a serious sleep disorder in which breathing repeatedly stops and starts.

Light therapy can reset your internal biological clock. Researchers at the University of Colorado at Boulder found that exposure to approximately 10,000 lux of bright light for 6.7 hours during the rising and descending phases of the cortisol rhythm reduced cortisol levels.[3]

Phosphatidylserine, mostly found in soy, might positively regulate sleep quality – and also preserve or increase brain functions.

Sleep during dark hours and make sure your bedroom is dark. Give your body a chance to activate melatonin, a hormone the brain produces in response to darkness. Reduce exposure to bright light after dark. Lower your lights. If you've got a lot of ambient light coming through the windows, invest in some blackout shades.

Keep your room cool.

Stop using your electronic devices a few hours before bedtime. Because of its wavelength, blue light from your devices disrupts healthy sleep. Blue-light-sensitive cells, known as intrinsically photosensitive retinal ganglion cells, or ipRGCs, tell the brain's "master clock" how much light there is in the environment. So, when you look at one of your brightly lit screens, these cells help set your internal clock for daytime-level alertness. Not good! Put your screens on night-mode and consider blue-light blocking glasses. To get seven-to-eight hours of sleep each night, keep those screens out of the bedroom.

Swear off caffeine, alcohol, heavy meals, and strenuous exercise close to bedtime. They all raise cortisol levels.

Expose yourself to natural light for at least 10 minutes right after waking up. This helps synchronize your circadian clock.

Blood sugar control

You know now that an **abnormal blood sugar level** will keep your stress high and keep perpetuating your cravings for unhealthy foods (see Chapter 8: "Cortisol and Weight Loss: Why So Many Diets Fail"). Candy bars, sugary drinks, and most commercial snacks are not your friend as they raise your cortisol and insulin levels. Makes sense since, cortisol is in charge of regulating your blood sugar levels (remember it is a gluco-corticoid). Fight back by eating at least 25-35 grams of high fiber foods (not supplements). Add in fermented foods, such as, yogurt, kefir, fermented cottage cheese, kimchi, vegetable brine drinks, and kombucha tea. All of these help increase your gut's microbial diversity.

Eat complex carbs in the right order (last) and never by themselves, since combining them with fats and proteins lowers their glycemic effect. A poor night sleep raises both cortisol and your blood sugar.

Drink apple cider vinegar. Well, not straight from the bottle. Add a few teaspoons to your shake, salad dressing, or pickles. A group of Iranian researchers found that consuming apple cider vinegar significantly decreased serum total cholesterol and fasting plasma glucose.[4] And exercise.

Chronic inflammation

You know that chronic inflammation triggers obesity, metabolic disorders, and abnormal gut permeability. Once again, you can control inflammation in your body by eating wholesome foods and exercising. Left unchecked, inflammation can contribute to a host of chronic diseases, such as heart disease, diabetes, obesity, cancer, and Alzheimer's disease, to name just a few of the top disabling conditions. Interactions between inflamed body tissue and the HPA axis kind of egg each other on, ultimately creating a vicious cycle of stress and activation.

We're encouraging you to practice time-restricted eating by instituting a schedule where you fast for 12-to-14 hours and limit your eating to a 10-hour window – without snacking. Researchers at the University of Florida - Gainesville found that the "metabolic switch from glucose to fatty acid-derived ketones represents an evolutionarily conserved trigger point that shifts metabolism from lipid/cholesterol synthesis and fat storage to mobilization of fat through fatty acid oxidation and fatty-acid derived ketones, which serve to preserve muscle mass and function."[5] Put more simply, intermittent fasting will bring down your insulin levels, reduce your body weight, and improve your body composition, which, in turn, will lower your cortisol.

What about breakfast? If you're stressed and feeling debilitated, it's best to make breakfast part of your meal plan. Researchers at the US Army Research Institute of Environmental Medicine did a study that showed "positive to neutral support" for eating breakfast, which led to "improvements in appetite control, satiety, and postprandial energy expenditure."[6] But more about that later.

Nutrition

The word "diet" alone could probably raise your cortisol levels! That's why we prefer to talk about a food plan. The operative word here is "plan." We understand that with all the forces in your life pulling you in different directions, planning out your meals, and your family's, can itself be a source of stress.

But nothing in life proceeds without a fair amount of planning, and your nutritional intake is no different. Tasty, unprocessed foods can protect your body from infections and diseases, such as heart disease, diabetes, and cancer. They can also improve your mood, energy, and focus. After all, food is information telling your genes what to do.

That brings us back to our old friend, cortisol. We still need to see much more research on the relationship between cortisol levels and food quality, but one significant study by New York University researchers found a link between low-quality foods high in sugar, salt, and fat content and an impaired hypothalamic-pituitary-adrenal (HPA) axis.[7] Indeed, the researchers found that high cortisol levels were associated with the consumption of certain meats, junk food, soda, fried foods, fast food, and simple carbohydrates in Type 2 Diabetes.[8] Another study by researchers at the University of Cincinnati links hyperactivity in the sympathetic nervous system (SNS) and the HPA axis with visceral obesity, or excess abdominal fat. Moreover, the aroused SNS and HPA spur the craving for comfort foods with low nutritive value.[9]

Meanwhile, a number of foods can help "relax" your cortisol levels. Many of them are part of the Mediterranean diet: fish, poultry, vegetables, fruits, whole grains and healthy fats. Indeed, the healthy fats – specifically food with omega-3 fatty acids – associated with this diet help reduce inflammation, and therefore, cortisol.[10] [11]

The best food for reducing inflammation is fish. If you are strictly vegetarian, you can find these "good fats" in avocados, olives, flaxseed, walnuts and MCT oils derived from coconut oil.

You can also get healthy fats from certain animal products, such as butter and ghee from grass-fed cows and goats, meat and dairy products from pastured animals, and free-range organic poultry.

No doubt, when we talk about fats of any kind, your mind can't help but go to cholesterol. It's true that high cholesterol will develop fatty deposits in your blood vessels, and when these deposits grow, blood has a hard time flowing through your arteries. If these deposits break free as clots, they can cause a heart attack or a stroke. That's why an adult should work to keep cholesterol below 200 mg/dL. Borderline high is 200 to 239 mg/dL.

But your body needs cholesterol too! Cholesterol that's less than 140 mg/dl is actually bad news for your steroid hormones. These include your sex hormones and your cortisol – all synthesized from cholesterol. So, no very low-fat diets.

Here's your reward: You can eat 80%-100% dark chocolate! It's rich in magnesium, which helps lower cortisol, and in polyphenols, organic compounds in plant-based foods that are full of antioxidants.

Now, we can't advocate "supplementing" your way out of high cortisol levels. Even the healthiest diet won't balance your cortisol levels without your commitment to sleep, exercise and a healthy mindset. But they nonetheless can be an important component of an overall food plan – especially when we know that the majority of Americans have inadequate intake of micronutrients, such as magnesium, Vitamins A, C, E, D and zinc, and are putting themselves at risk for a compromised immune system.[12]

Let's look at some of the most significant – and easily obtainable – nutritional supplements that will supply the adrenal glands with the building blocks to produce steroid hormones.

Vitamin C. Researchers at the University of Alabama - Huntsville found that large doses of Vitamin C can prevent illness by alleviating the body's normal response to stress.[13] The adrenal gland is among the organs with the highest concentration of Vitamin C in the body. Eskimos – the indigenous peoples of eastern Siberia and Alaska – don't get scurvy, a disease caused by Vitamin C deficiency, because they eat the adrenal glands of their fish and seal catch.

Vitamin B. The B vitamins help regulate your production of cortisol and they are in greater demand when you're under chronic stress. Researchers at the Swinburne University of Technology in Australia found that their treatment groups receiving complex Vitamin B reported significantly lower personal strain and a reduction in confusion and depressed/dejected mood after 12 weeks.[14] B vitamins are cofactors in the synthesis of hormones and neurotransmitters, and the right amount, especially of Vitamin B12, is essential for the healthy functioning of adrenal hormones.[15] We recommend a good B complex vitamin, as well as B5 and B6. Note that bananas, rich in Vitamin B6, are a great source for maintaining proper adrenal gland function.

Calcium. Researchers at Harvard University and Brigham and Women's Hospital have found evidence that the bidirectional relationships between adrenal- and calcium-regulating systems promote cardiovascular and bone health.[16]

Magnesium. Researchers at the Institute of Pharmacy and the University of Innsbruck, Austria, found that magnesium deficiencies could provoke anxiety-like behavior and perturbed HPA function in a series of tests on laboratory mice.[17] (Some animal and clinical studies suggest complementary effects of magnesium and high-dose pyridoxine (vitamin B6) on stress reduction.[18]

Zinc. Researchers at the University of Shizuoka in Japan have observed that zinc deficiency causes abnormal glucocorticoid secretion from the adrenal cortex.[19] They learned further that zinc deficiency elicits neuropsychological symptoms and affects cognitive performance. While zinc homeostasis in the brain is not easily disrupted by a dietary zinc deficiency, it's certainly worth maintaining healthy zinc levels in your body by taking a zinc supplement or by upping your consumption of beans, nuts, crab, lobster, whole grains, and low-fat dairy products.[20]

Potassium and Sodium. An appropriate amount of potassium and sodium are crucial for maintaining high-functioning adrenal glands. An imbalance leads to salt cravings – and, more seriously, low body fluid and low blood pressure. If you have a low cortisol number, you'll want to take some sea salt in the morning. Salted vegetable juices with water are also a good option. (Fruit and fruit drinks are not.) Researchers have observed an increased potassium to sodium ratio in patients with poorly functioning adrenals.

We know our basic recommendation looks easy on paper:

Find a diet that's appropriate for your own biology and your goals. Eat sufficient calories by focusing on pastured or wild caught protein sources, fiber-rich and fermented foods, and unprocessed foods – mostly plants.

We also know that changing your diet, probably one you've stuck with since childhood, is like turning a battleship around. If you can't find friends or other people in your community as a healthy food support group, look online for virtual support. Meetup, for example, offers healthy eating groups all around the US, addressing everything from ayurveda (a system of medicine that believes disease is caused by an imbalance or stress in a person's consciousness) to "veggification" (OK, that's an invented word).

Exercise

We've already talked about elite athletes and the heights they push themselves to. We've talked about hormetic stress, which shocks your body into adapting rapidly to stressful events. Admittedly, both of these approaches to exercise are on the outer edges of normal. What you want is to incorporate an exercise plan into your daily routine. Most people can handle brisk walking, jogging, swimming, yoga, Pilates, and/or strength-training.

We don't recommend running a marathon or any other extreme physical exertion when you have HPA axis dysregulation. It can deplete the body and lead to immunosuppression.[21]

Time of day is significant. It's better to exercise in the morning than in the evening. A study led by researchers at the University of North Carolina-Chapel Hill found that early-in-the-day exercisers lost significantly more weight compared with late-in-the-day exercisers.[22] And as we said earlier, it's best to avoid strenuous exercise in the hours before bedtime: Late-in-the-day exercise raises your cortisol levels.

Let's say you eat well, exercise, and sleep eight hours at night. Chances are good that you're still going to encounter stress. You can prepare for stress by taking action against it when it comes. We've quantified three ways of preparing for it

2) Support your HPA axis

Measure cortisol to assess the status of your HPA axis. We'll say this loud and proud from cover to cover. Pardigm.com will be ready to support you in 2023.

Adaptogens

To promote brain and HPA axis health, remove modifiable stressors (see above) and incorporate adaptogens into your food plan.

Adaptogens are plants and mushrooms that help your body respond appropriately to stress, anxiety, and fatigue. They frequently come in tincture or capsule form, and are easy to add to shakes, tea, and soups. While adaptogens have not been accepted as conventional therapies in western medicine, they are known to "either reduce stress reactions in the alarm phase or retard/prevent the exhaustion phase and thus provide a certain degree of protection against long-term stress."[23] Many adaptogens have been used for thousands of years all over the globe.

A few of the popular adaptogens that can help balance cortisol levels and boost HPA axis functionality are :

Ashwagandha. Botanically known as *Withania somnifera*, this herb has a prominent place in ayurvedic medicine. "Ashwagandha" comes from the Sanskrit for "horse-like smell," and, well, the herb takes a little getting used to. The benefits, however, make a strong case for tolerating the taste and smell: In a study by researchers at Asha Hospital in Hyderabad, study subjects who took ashwagandha to reduce their stress symptoms saw a 27.9% reduction in their cortisol levels. A placebo-control group saw only a 7.9% reduction. The researchers concluded that individuals who use high-concentration full-spectrum ashwagandha root extract can potentially realize improvements in their neurological, immune, energy-production, endocrine, and reproductive systems.[24]

Rhodiola rosea*.* A review study by Australian and Swedish researchers found that *Rhodiola* preparations used by various body organs, tissues, cells, and enzymes exhibited "neuroprotective, cardioprotective, anti-fatigue, antidepressive, anxiolytic, nootropic, life-span increasing effects, and central nervous system (CNS) stimulating activity."[25] Some clinical trials showed that this herb reduced burnout in patients with so-called "fatigue syndrome."[26] Several mechanisms contributing to *Rhodiola's* positive effects on mild depression and generalized anxiety include interactions with the HPA axis to reduce cortisol levels.[27]

Ginseng. Found in central and eastern North America, Manchuria, Japan, and Korea, the ginseng herb has a long-time favorable reputation for combatting stress, enhancing the central and immune systems, fending off chronic disease states, and inhibiting the aging process. Canadian researchers studied whether the herb had specific toxic and healthful effects on humans, animals, and *in vitro* subjects. The researchers found that ginseng appeared to bring about changes in circulating levels of adrenocorticotrophin (ACTH), hormone and corticosterone concentrations.[28] They noted too, that ginseng's tendency to produce "ergogenic," or enhanced physical performance, may be due to improved activity of the "pituitary-adrenal axis."

Phellodendron amurense*.* More popularly known as relora, this herb has traditionally been used to reduce stress and anxiety – particularly among competitive athletes. A study by Utah-based researchers showed that "daily supplementation with a combination of magnolia bark extract and *Phellodendron* bark extract (Relora®) reduces cortisol exposure and perceived daily stress, while improving a variety of mood state parameters, including lower fatigue and higher vigor." Over the course of a 4-week Relora® supplementation period, the researchers found that "salivary cortisol exposure was significantly lower (−18%) in the Relora® group.[29]

Keep your adrenals healthy

Adrenals like routine and order. Good nutrition, good sleep, and good exercise are the holy trinity of adrenal support. Supplement your health with vitamins and minerals that you might be missing. Speak with your practitioner about taking glandulars (animal source adrenal extracts) or hormonal supplements like hydrocortisone, DHEA, progesterone and/or pregnenolone to re-establish neurotransmitter and hormonal balance. It's not safe to take any of these without guidance from a knowledgeable professional.

Change the way target tissues respond to cortisol. We want to do this by affecting the enzymes that metabolize cortisol. Consuming licorice root extract is a great way to accomplish this – it inhibits 11betaHSD2 – and supports cortisol levels when they are low; if you take it, watch for elevated blood pressure.

3) Become resilient to stress

Build metabolic flexibility – the ability to respond to changes in metabolic demand – by exercising and working the heart.[30]

We believe you can do this by practicing hormesis: a series of short, intermittent bursts of certain stressors that trigger a cascade of cellular processes intended to initiate cellular repair mechanisms, making you more resilient to physical and mental stress in the future and slowing aging.

We also believe you can build mental resilience by embracing a "stress-is-enhancing" mindset (see Chapter 10: "Scientific Breakthrough: Mindset Controls Cortisol"). Mindset, rigorously studied by Dr. Alia Crum at the Stanford Mind and Body Lab, encompasses the "core assumptions we make about the things and processes in the world that orient us to a particular set of expectations, explanations, and goals."[31] Mindsets can change how we see ourselves, our community, and our interpersonal relationships. Indeed, much of Dr. Crum's work is built on the premise that "intelligence is malleable"[32] in the face of stress, conflict, and ever-changing environmental conditions. We found it so important, we dedicated a whole chapter to it.

Should you skip breakfast?

By: Jessica Cohn-Kleinberg

Let's take a deeper dive. We've all heard it before: "Breakfast is the most important meal of the day." That belief has been pushed by the breakfast industry for a century, urging consumers to load up on cereal, bacon and orange juice at the grocery store.

Yet, science is still debating breakfast — not only how it affects our health and weight, but if it's even necessary.

Should you skip your next breakfast?

The choice comes down to your diet and individual health needs. To make the most informed decision, though, it's important to understand the history of breakfast and how skipping your morning meal can impact your body.

"Breakfast is the most important meal of the day" hasn't been common wisdom for terribly long. In fact, prior to the seventeenth century, breakfast was largely frowned upon. The Romans only believed in eating one large meal a day, a practice that influenced eating habits long after. Indeed, in the Middle Ages, many people didn't eat before morning mass.

Then, around the seventeenth century, breakfast came into vogue. The wealthy started to enjoy coffee, tea, and easy-to-prepare foods, such as scrambled eggs. In the middle of the century, they even began adding breakfast rooms into their homes.

It wasn't until 1917, however, that dietitian Lenna Cooper suggested that breakfast was the most important meal of the day. She detailed her argument in an article for *Good Health* magazine, which was published by a sanitarium run by, none other than, Dr. John Harvey Kellogg.

Yes, the same Kellogg who, with his brother, invented and mass-marketed the world's first corn flakes. Dr. Kellogg also edited *Good Health* magazine.

Marketing teams did wonders for breakfast's reputation in the early twentieth century. In the 1920s, for example, the Beech-Nut Packing company hired Edward Bernays, known as the father of public relations, to sell bacon. Bernays went to work. First, he managed to get a doctor to agree that bacon and eggs were healthier options for breakfast. He then got some 5,000 doctors to sign a petition making this claim. Finally, he worked with newspapers to publish the results as if they were part of a scientific study. This marketing gambit gave fuel to the rising belief that eating breakfast was a medical necessity.

It wasn't until 1944, though, that breakfast cemented its place as the day's most important meal. That's when Grape-Nuts, a breakfast cereal, launched the campaign: "Eat a Good Breakfast — Do a Better Job." As part of this promotion, Grape-Nuts handed out pamphlets and blared radio ads proclaiming: "Nutrition experts say breakfast is the most important meal of the day."

The rest, as they say, is history.

Many health professionals are still in favor of eating breakfast. It's been the prevailing recommendation for the past century, after all. And with some good reasons.

Eating breakfast may help with weight control. While debated, some studies point to eating breakfast as a method of weight control, because it can help with stabilizing your internal clock, as well as curtailing appetite and snacking later in the day.

In one 2018 review of breakfast consumption and weight management published in *Advanced Nutrition*, researchers found positive-to-neutral support for using breakfast to control appetite. Ultimately, they said it can come down to what you're eating. Meals with more protein, solid food and calories (greater than 350 calories) helped control appetite when compared to skipping breakfast.

Eating breakfast can make you feel better. If you eat dinner between 6 and 8 PM. and then wait until lunch to eat again, that's a lot of time without any external fuel. Some people will experience dips in blood sugar, dizziness, headaches and difficulty concentrating when they wait too long to eat.

Healthy blood sugar levels are, of course, vital to your health. A review in 2016 found that eating breakfast improved glucose and insulin responses throughout the day in comparison to skipping breakfast, although the exact foods played a role. A comparable study highlighted the value of early time-restricted eating in which participants consumed meals during daylight hours. Think between 8 AM and 2 PM. It found that early eating improved 24-

hour glucose levels, helped stabilize circadian rhythms — and may even have anti-aging effects, along with other benefits.

Skipping breakfast has also been linked to an increased risk of type 2 diabetes, in which your body isn't able to use insulin to store glucose (blood sugar) properly. This causes your blood sugar levels to build up and can lead to a number of serious health complications.

Eating breakfast can also boost your overall sense of wellbeing. One study found that a small breakfast eaten before exercising can benefit your mood afterward.

The bonus? We tend to make healthier food choices when we're happy, according to researchers in the US and South Korea. The feel-good feeling you have after breakfast could arguably lead to a better diet.

Your body can log a skipped breakfast as a stressful event. When you skip your morning meal, it could disrupt your body's internal clock. Studies show that meals help synchronize our clocks, including how we release hormones and metabolize fat, so unusual eating times may result in unhealthy outcomes.

In fact, this disruption may be why your body sees fasting as a stressful event. As a 2015 study found, skipping breakfast is linked to increased concentrations of cortisol. As we've seen, cortisol imbalances can lead to a number of health risks, including weight gain, diabetes and other conditions.

Many people don't have an appetite for breakfast. Indeed, fasting, which we talked about in Chapter 8, has become a popular topic in wellness circles. Some research backs up the health benefits.

Skipping breakfast can help with weight control. In a 2019 meta-analysis of 13 randomized controlled trials, researchers found a small difference in weight, favoring participants who skipped breakfast. This study suggests that eating breakfast might not be a good strategy for weight loss and could actually cause weight gain.

Another nutrition study examined 17 healthy adults who skipped breakfast and found people can burn more calories on days they skip the meal. They noted, however, this may increase inflammation. And because chronic inflammation can affect insulin sensitivity, it's possible that skipping breakfast could contribute to "metabolic impairment" — a disorder that could potentially raise the risk for obesity and type 2 diabetes.

Further studies, however, are needed. Keep in mind that the researchers only measured inflammation levels after lunch, so skipping breakfast could simply increase inflammation at lunchtime while decreasing it during other periods.

The study also followed adults across three days, so the results say nothing about the health effects of regularly skipping breakfast.

Skipping breakfast is a "hormetic stress" event that can benefit your health. Short bursts of pressure on the body, such as intermittent fasting or caloric restriction, may provide the type of stressful event that kicks off an adaptive response. This "hormesis" can actually increase your resilience to stress down the line.

Hormetic stress experts theorize that we adapted to common stressors such as food scarcity as we evolved — so those triggers "became integral parts of who we are," according to researchers in The Netherlands.

In two observational nutrition studies, for example, intermittent fasting was linked to reduced instances of coronary artery disease and diabetes. And a 2017 Singapore-based review underscored that it can extend lifespan and aid in the fight against cardiovascular and neurodegenerative diseases (think Alzheimer's and Parkinson's) in animals. It can even slow the progression of cancer in those models.

Keep in mind: As with other forms of hormetic stress, intermittent fasting is not for everyone. People with medical conditions, the elderly, and pregnant women, to name a few, may be at risk. Remember to practice any caloric restriction with the oversight of a healthcare professional.

Skipping breakfast can cut out the sugar and refined carbs found in typical dishes. Sugary breakfast cereals are a classic. Although some say a healthy serving shouldn't go over 10 grams of sugar, the average box of cereal can contain 19.8 grams of sugar for every serving. Just think of the other breakfast staples that contain sugar: muffins, yogurt with fruit, orange juice, toast with jam, pancakes with syrup. The list goes on.

It's inescapable: All too many breakfast foods in the western diet are packed with too much sugar, and with too many processed and refined carbohydrates. The draw: These dishes are convenient. Most don't need to be cooked or cooked for long. And they don't go bad quickly. How could they, with preservative ingredients such as sugar, corn syrup, dextrose, and malt flavor?

Think of jammy toast or cereal. These typical breakfast options cut down on time when you're rushing out the door. Unfortunately, they just aren't healthy. They spike your glucose, which will spike your insulin. Skipping breakfast can be the healthier option when you're eating these types of processed foods.

In a 2018 study of 527 adolescents, breakfast skippers showed better health-related quality of life and lower levels of stress and depression than breakfast eaters who ate a poor or very poor quality breakfast.

Researchers continue to debate the merits of eating breakfast, but one thing is clear: The type of food you eat matters.

While we continue to learn more about how our meals affect

our health, it's a good bet to lean into a breakfast made up of a quality protein source, fiber-rich vegetables and healthy fats.

If it's too difficult to make in the morning, remember that for some people, skipping breakfast may be fine.

For thousands of years, the cortisol awakening response has been our natural breakfast, pushing glucose into our bloodstream and getting us ready for the day. So there doesn't seem to be a need to add even more food. If you want to lose weight and improve your metabolic health, you might want to limit the insulin spikes per day. Managing your stress and skipping breakfast can be a good test. Listen to your body and see if it benefits you.

Skipping breakfast is not for everyone.

If you are already stressed and struggling with imbalanced cortisol levels, you might not want to push yourself by adding the additional stressor of skipping breakfast. In that case, it's better to eat a breakfast rich in proteins, fiber, and good fats within 30 to 60 minutes after waking up.

Know that if you're severely stressed, have unstable blood sugar levels or take medicines affecting your blood sugar, have other medical considerations, or if your body is not used to ketosis — brought on by a low-carb, high-protein, fat-burning diet — skipping breakfast and impacting your glucose levels should be done under medical supervision, if done at all.

Listen to your body. Listen to your doctor. Then make a decision that meets your health needs and goals. At the end of the day, our bodies are unique, complicated machines that require individually tailored solutions. That's the path to true health care.

Hot Saunas and Hormetic Stress: A New Way to Fight Anxiety?

By: Jessica Cohn-Kleinberg

You can tackle your stress.

By adding more stress to your life.

A paradox? Maybe, but a growing body of research explores the benefits of exposing your body to short bursts of pressure, or hormetic stress. Some studies suggest this can help prepare you emotionally, mentally and physically for life's tough times.

You may already be familiar with hormetic stress in the form of high-intensity interval training, or HIIT. You dive into a short explosive exercise that raises your heart rate and then you stop to recover for a very brief period. You rinse-and-repeat to aid in stress resistance.[33]

Hot saunas and intermittent fasting are also examples of hormetic stress.[34] These practices create brief surges in your biological stress response, followed by a type of recovery you might otherwise have a hard time managing. And yet, it can help you, body and mind, become more resilient.

Let's look at two things: First, how can these types of activities strengthen your stress response? Second, what are the possible risks?

When you're stressed physically or mentally, your internal alarm system flips into "on" mode. Suddenly, your adrenal glands produce hormones, such as cortisol, to help you face the threat. This quick hormonal burst can raise your blood pressure, heart rate, blood sugar and more, before bringing you back to your baseline — all with the goal of helping you respond to the stressor in your environment.

However, the "flight, fight, freeze or fawn" response,[35] was not built for the unique problems of modern-day life. Most of our stressors are difficult to fight off without the right tools and nearly impossible to flee. Just worrying can set off a hormonal response. Consequently, your "alarm system" is stuck in "on" mode, and you're a candidate for chronic stress.

Interestingly, hormetic stress is a category of acute, or short-term, stress. It stands to reason that it's not chronic because it rapidly returns you to a desired state of homeostasis — your baseline. The goal of hormetic stress is to shock you biologically into adapting quickly to a stressful event. It's meant to condition your stress response by building up your resiliency.

Timing is a key component of hormetic stress. The quick stressful event should be mild or moderate, followed by a swift recovery. "The exact timing of stressor exposure is an important determinant of a hormetic or pre-conditioning effect, as some stressors lead to sensitization across stressors, rather than habituation."[36]

A recent study examined the benefits of exposing mice to hormetic stress.[37] Researchers found that a quick stressor — restraint for five minutes each day — could reverse depressive-like behavior over two weeks. However, when restrained longer, say, for 15 minutes, the benefits of this short-term stress were not sustained.

Hormetic stress may even go beyond building resiliency or reversing depression. Some researchers in the field of gero-science, or the biological processes of aging, suggest it could slow the aging process.[38]

Hormetic-stress activities can come with medical concerns, particularly for people who fall into risk-sensitive categories. That's why it's important to consult your healthcare provider practitioner before attempting any new activity. With that in mind, here are four examples of hormetic stress, along with some associated risks.

Vigorous Breathing Exercises: Elissa Epel,[39] professor of psychiatry at the University of California, is leading a study[40] that asks if short-term hormetic stress interventions make us more resilient. Her team will focus on the physiological and mood effects of three types of controlled stress: a meditation practice, intense exercise and hypoxic breathing — a practice developed by Wim Hof, an extreme athlete known for his ability to withstand extreme cold.

Hypoxia is a condition in which the body's tissues do not get sufficient oxygen. Hypoxic breathing is a practice, developed by extreme athlete Wim Hof, that challenges your body to adapt to lower levels of oxygen. It's basically breath control. He and other researchers have long detailed how sublethal hypoxic events, or "preconditioning," "can improve the tolerance of not only cells or tissues, but also entire organs and even the organism itself, to subsequent hypoxia."[41]

Hof has developed a method for tapping into preconditioning. His hypoxic breathing practice includes 30 to 40 deep, intense breaths followed by an extended exhale and one more breath held at full capacity for 15 seconds. You can repeat this cycle three to four times.

If you're doing a double-take, you're not alone! The technique is considered controversial. After all, you're denying yourself oxygen. Wim Hof's website advises this can lead to lightheadedness and a tingling sensation in your fingers. It also warns that it could affect motor control and, in rare cases, cause loss of consciousness. The website does not recommend the practice for people who have serious health conditions, such as high blood pressure, heart disease, epilepsy and more.

Exposure to Extreme Temperatures: Another form of hormetic stress includes exposure to extreme hot or cold temperatures. In 2015 a multinational research team examined 2,315 Finnish men to study the impact on them of extreme hot or cold temperatures.[42] The men who enjoyed going to the sauna two or three times a week for 20 minutes were 23% less likely to die of cardiovascular disease than those who visited the sauna once a week. The more extreme sauna users, who went four to seven times a week, were 48% less likely to die.

Another case[43] showed extreme cold exposure (along with hypoxic breathing exercises) significantly increased adrenaline production. It underscored how acute stressors boost autonomic activity, expedite immune cell proliferation and differentiation, and stimulate the immune system's anti-inflammatory response.

Think of it this way: Cold exposure can give a jolt to your cardiovascular system by constricting blood vessels, causing a workout for your heart, and possibly pre-conditioning you against future stressors.

One method of doing this is with showering in cold water for as long as you can take, according to Mr. Hof. This could start at 15 seconds then get bumped up as tolerance grows.

Intense Bursts of Activity: Next we have high-intensity interval training, also known as HIIT. Higher intensity exercise can increase your cortisol, but it can suppress your cortisol response to future stressors.[44]

It makes sense: Cortisol initially rises to manage your body's growth as you tackle the stressful exercise. But your system can adapt, muting your future hormonal response and building your resiliency. That comes with a host of potential health implications for dealing with chronic stress.

In one study[45] published in 2021, researchers studied the effects of HIIT and moderate-intensity training (MIT) on anxiety, depression, stress and resiliency during lockdown. Both exercises significantly lowered stress, anxiety, and depression levels and even increased resilience. Yet HIIT was more effective at reducing depression than MIT.

Dietary Disruptions: Finally, we come to diet. Intermittent fasting or caloric restriction may also provide the type of stressful event that kicks off an adaptive response, increasing your resilience to stress down the line. After all, hormetic stress experts theorize that we adapted to common stressors such as food scarcity as we evolved — so those triggers "became integral parts of who we are."[46]

For example, in two observational studies,[47] intermittent fasting was linked to reduced instances of coronary artery disease and diabetes. And one 2017 review[48] underscored that it can extend lifespan and aid in the fight against cardiovascular and neurodegenerative diseases (think Alzheimer's and Parkinson's) in animals. It can even slow the progression of cancer in those models.

But remember: As with other forms of hormetic stress, doctors are concerned about possible risks, especially for those with medical conditions or who are elderly or pregnant.

Interestingly, phytochemicals or "plant chemicals" such as polyphenols, alkaloids and terpenoids found in plants and fungi also cause nutritional hormesis — meaning ingesting them can create low-level stress in your body. As a result, they can trigger the same adaptive response as caloric restriction, fasting and exercise.[49]

As mentioned in a 2018 review, phytochemicals acting via hormetic stress, can potentially protect "against cancer, neurodegenerative diseases, cardiovascular diseases, inflammatory and immune diseases by acting on multiple stress-response pathways."[50]

Ultimately, this body of research continues to expand. But hormetic stress is a good reminder that not all stress is bad for your health. And that humans are more resilient than you might think.

———

A few other stress-management hacks to have up your sleeve :

Neuroscientist Andrew Huberman, who studies the brain's function, plasticity and recovery and the visual system involvement in stress response at Stanford University's Huberman Lab,

RECOMMENDATIONS: HOW TO KEEP YOUR CORTISOL LEVELS BA...

offers up a tactical means of ameliorating burnout and its negative impact on your body and mind. He calls it the physiological sigh.

It's easy to do. And it works.

"You can quickly calm the body down by doing this double-inhale, long-exhale practice," he says. "Typically the rapid inhales are done though the nose, the exhale through the mouth. Stress researchers have known about the physiological sigh since the 1930s. It's the fastest real-time tool we have for taking down one's state of alertness."

Huberman says the technique works because you are "controlling" the mind with your body, not with your mind. "Telling yourself, "Don't stress, don't stress, calm down, calm down," rarely works when you're in the midst of a stressful situation," he says. "The physiological sigh is effective because you're doing something purely mechanical. Once you manage your breathing like this, the mind has a chance to relax."

Practice the physiological sigh before you go to work, before you step into a meeting, before you answer the phone call of a difficult colleague. The physiological sigh slows the heart rate and calms the fight-or-flight response. It helps us regain control of a moment that feels as if it's spinning out of control. Repeat as much as necessary whenever you feel overwhelmed by workplace stress. The science shows it should bring you some relief.

Psychiatrist David Spiegel, who is head of the Stanford Center on Stress and Health,[51] has been studying pain control, psychoneuroendocrinology, sleep and hypnosis for over 40 years. He doesn't see hypnosis as a form of therapy, but as a therapeutic technique that can be used as an adjunct to other therapies. If you are one of the lucky hypnotizable ones – he recommends a test to check for that[52]– check out the self-hypnosis app, Reveri, and try the short 5-10 minutes practices to help you deal with stress.

Takeaways

- It's easier to fix your cortisol imbalance than to live with its long-term consequences.

- Abnormal cortisol patterns, which reflect HPA axis dysregulation, can be fixed by changing lifestyle habits.

- Measure and follow your cortisol levels if they're abnormal.

- Keep mindset in mind! It's not stress, it's your response to it.

For More Information

Sign up, so you can be the first to know when test strips become available. Visit www.masterhormone.com.

Investors or business partners are invited to drop us a note at info@pardigm.com.

Media requests should be sent to media@pardigm.com.

It's amazing how few people know about cortisol and how it shapes our lives. Help us get the word out. Share what you've learned from this book with your physician, family, and friends. Let's get everybody educated about the power of cortisol!

Erratum

We've done our best to provide you with the latest in cortisol research, but with the rapid pace of technological development, our book runs the risk of becoming outdated in various particulars. We apologize for any unintentional errors. We know we can't make an omelet without breaking some eggs, so we've included an erratum with updates and insights at www.masterhormone.com.

Pardigm.com Intro

Pardigm, Inc. is a well-funded Silicon Valley biotech startup founded by mobile & AI pioneer Wibe Wagemans. It is the first company to offer a real-time, quantitative test to measure cortisol, thereby eliminating the need for expensive lab intervention. Pardigm's cortisol- measuring technology will help the world tackle stress, the health epidemic of the 21st century, according to the World Health Organization.

For decades, scientists have been trying to measure cortisol in a scalable way. Pardigm.com's breakthrough technology, using Computer Vision and Deep Learning (CVDL) technologies, will let anyone with a smartphone camera[1] capture and receive test results instantly.

Pardigm.com's technology is a wellness product and does not diagnose, treat, cure, or prevent any disease or health condition. Our content is for informational and educational purposes only, and does not substitute for medical advice or consultations with healthcare professionals.

NOTES

AN INVITATION

1. https://www.sciencedirect.com/science/article/pii/S235228952100028X
2. https://www.sciencedaily.com/releases/2009/12/091209114150.htm#:~:text=A%20first%2Dof%2Dits%2D,between%2050%20and%201532%20A.D.&text=Recent%20studies%20show%20that%20one,number%20is%20on%20the%20rise
3. A study of baleen whale cortisol levels reveals strikingly similar observations. Techniques involving baleen earplugs – historically investigated as a metric for aging – combine age estimates with cortisol measurements to assess the impact of "anthropogenic pressures," such as whale hunts and navy boats, on whales. Researchers conclude that baleen whales exhibit elevated cortisol levels in response to disturbances in their environment provoked by human beings.
4. https://www.pardigm.com/
5. We'll talk more about this baseline, or visual representation of your test results, in Chapter 2.

FOREWORD

1. https://youtu.be/3rcjKLes1GA?t=1816
2. Genomics Collaborative and Skolar were each later acquired by other life sciences companies.
3. https://journals.sagepub.com/doi/epub/10.1177/0004563216687335

1. GET TO KNOW US BECAUSE WE WANT TO KNOW YOU

1. https://pubmed.ncbi.nlm.nih.gov/29909048/
2. https://www.ncbi.nlm.nih.gov/pmc/articles/PMC5414803/#B177
3. https://pubmed.ncbi.nlm.nih.gov/34650525/
4. https://www.ninds.nih.gov/news-events/press-releases/gut-trains-immune-system-protect-brain
5. Clow A, Smyth N. Salivary cortisol as a non-invasive window on the brain. Int Rev Neurobiol. 2020;150:1-16. doi: 10.1016/bs.irn.2019.12.003. Epub 2020 Jan 10. PMID: 32204827.
6. https://www.nejm.org/doi/Physician Burnout, Interrupted | NEJM-full/10.1056/NEJMp2003149

NOTES

7. https://www.medscape.com/slideshow/2022-physician-suicide-report-6014970#2
8. https://www.ncbi.nlm.nih.gov/pmc/articles/PMC4997656/
9. https://www.proquest.com/docview/939525985?pq-origsite=gscholar&fromopenview=true
10. https://journals.lww.com/psychosomaticmedicine/Abstract/2000/09000/Stress_and_Body_Shape__Stress_Induced_Cortisol.5.aspx
11. https://www.ncbi.nlm.nih.gov/pmc/articles/PMC6758130/#B24
12. https://hbr.org/2015/09/stress-can-be-a-good-thing-if-you-know-how-to-use-it
13. Association of Diurnal Patterns in Salivary Cortisol with All-Cause and Cardiovascular Mortality: Findings from the Whitehall II Study | The Journal of Clinical Endocrinology & Metabolism
    8.Urinary cortisol and six-year risk of all-cause and cardiovascular mortality
14. https://www.goodrx.com/drug-guide
15. Telomeres are a protective casing at the end of a strand of DNA. When the telomere is too diminished, the cell often dies or becomes pro-inflammatory.
16. https://link.springer.com/article/10.14310/horm.2002.1217
17. https://www.ncbi.nlm.nih.gov/pmc/articles/PMC6450740/
18. https://www.nature.com/articles/s41598-022-14905-4
19. https://pubmed.ncbi.nlm.nih.gov/24833580/
20. https://pubmed.ncbi.nlm.nih.gov/15574496/
21. https://www.ncbi.nlm.nih.gov/pmc/articles/PMC2830080/
22. https://www.nature.com/articles/s41398-021-01550-0
23. https://pubmed.ncbi.nlm.nih.gov/33554551/
    This review summarizes and critically evaluates the published approaches and recent trends in techniques used for the determination of uric acid (UA) in saliva. UA is the final product of purine nucleotide catabolism in humans. Previous studies reported correlation between UA concentrations detected in saliva and in the blood. The evaluation of salivary UA levels can contribute to non-invasive diagnosis of many serious diseases. Increased salivary uric acid concentration is associated with cancer, HIV, gout, and hypertension. In contrast, low uric acid levels are associated with Alzheimer disease, progression of multiple sclerosis, and mild cognitive impairment.
24. https://www.pardigm.com/white-paper

2. WHY YOU SHOULD MEASURE YOUR CORTISOL LEVELS

1. https://en.wikipedia.org/wiki/Goldilocks_principle
2. https://www.ncbi.nlm.nih.gov/pmc/articles/PMC5868606/
3. More info about balancing your cortisol diurnal pattern at www.pardigm.com.
4. For science geeks and health professionals, we recommend an excellent book on Stress and the HPA axis by Thomas G. Guilliams, PhD. https://www.

NOTES

pointinstitute.org/product/the-role-of-stress-and-the-hpa-axis-in-chronic-disease-management-second-edition/

5. Melatonin is a neurohormone produced in the pineal gland of the brain, which follows a diurnal pattern opposite to cortisol. It is intimately involved in the body's circadian rhythm, along with cortisol.
6. Electronic screens emit blue light, a color likely to cause damage when absorbed by various cells in the body. For one, it blocks a hormone called melatonin that helps you fall asleep. Using your screens at night will keep you from getting drowsy. It'll take you longer to fall asleep and stay asleep.
7. https://psycnet.apa.org/record/2015-23511-001
8. https://www.sciencedirect.com/science/article/abs/pii/S0735109722049944
9. https://www.ncbi.nlm.nih.gov/pmc/articles/PMC5635140/
10. https://pubmed.ncbi.nlm.nih.gov/27262888/
11. Sleeping in a climate-controlled room can improve the quality of your sleep. That's because our body temperature drops at night. The metabolism rate slows down and we spend less energy during sleep. Hence, the importance of not getting overheated.
12. https://pubmed.ncbi.nlm.nih.gov/6316831/#:~:text=The%20relationship%20between%20salivary%20and,much%20less%20than%205%20minutes
13. https://www.uptodate.com/contents/measurement-of-cortisol-in-serum-and-saliva
14. https://pubmed.ncbi.nlm.nih.gov/28068807/
15. https://read.qxmd.com/read/18280810/advantage-of-salivary-cortisol-measurements-in-the-diagnosis-of-glucocorticoid-related-disorders
16. https://www.pointinstitute.org/product/the-role-of-stress-and-the-hpa-axis-in-chronic-disease-management-second-edition/
17. Theoretically, if you were to check your cortisol continuously, the curve in each cortisol iteration (see figures above) would look more like a jagged line due to its normal pulsatile secretion pattern. This jagged line would reflect the amount of stress you feel, the nutritiousness of the food you just ate, and/or the presence of alcohol or caffeine in your system. Indeed, cortisol is so sensitive to environmental change that even a loud noise on the street can send it into high gear and influence the shape of the diurnal cortisol curve.
18. https://academic.oup.com/jamia/article/26/2/106/5230918
19. https://www.google.com/url?q=https://www.fda.gov/science-research/about-science-research-fda/biomarkers-fda&sa=D&source=docs&ust=1660677725182409&usg=AOvVaw1a3OLcZAToc6qlBgoCv9Sf
20. https://www.volkskrant.nl/wetenschap/een-hormoontest-leert-u-snel-hoe-gestrest-u-bent-volgens-de-aanbieders-maar-is-bij-stress-meten-ook-weten~beb41d10/
21. www.pardigm.com
22. pardigm.com

NOTES

3. HOW MONITORING CORTISOL CAN HELP MANAGE BURNOUT, STRESS AND MENTAL DISORDERS

1. The statistic comes from the World Economic Forum. https://start.askwonder.com/insights/want-help-gather-intelligence-economy-around-burnout-nxmepgr63#
2. https://pubmed.ncbi.nlm.nih.gov/25433974/
3. The term "vicarious traumatization" was coined by psychoanalysts Lisa McCann and Laurie Anne Pearlman.
4. "Compassion fatigue: Coping with secondary traumatic stress disorder in those who treat the traumatized," https://psycnet.apa.org/record/1995-97891-000
5. https://www.ncbi.nlm.nih.gov/pmc/articles/PMC6002544/
6. https://www.ncbi.nlm.nih.gov/pmc/articles/PMC4867107/
7. https://pubmed.ncbi.nlm.nih.gov/8675562/
8. https://www.ncbi.nlm.nih.gov/pmc/articles/PMC6002544/
9. "Atypical Depression and Non-Atypical Depression: Is HPA Axis Function a Biomarker? A Systemic Review," https://www.researchgate.net/publication/320349625_Atypical_Depression_and_Non-Atypical_Depression_Is_HPA_Axis_Function_a_Biomarker_A_Systematic_Review
10. https://www.cambridge.org/core/journals/the-british-journal-of-psychiatry/article/prednisolone-suppression-test-in-depression-prospective-study-of-the-role-of-hpa-axis-dysfunction-in-treatment-resistance/A7BA9E15E5769FA473C118A3E62C0184
11. A concept related to the British neuroscientist Joe Herbert's ideas about early adversity
12. https://pubmed.ncbi.nlm.nih.gov/29150144/
13. Sapolsky describes cortisol effects as being permissive, stimulating, or suppressive for an ongoing stress-response or preparative for a subsequent stressor, depending on the timing and duration of stress https://academic.oup.com/edrv/article/21/1/55/2423840
14. This affirmation was voiced by Stuart Smiley, a character invented by Al Franken for "Saturday Night Live," a popular U.S. television show.
15. https://www.pnas.org/doi/abs/10.1073/pnas.0409174102
16. https://www.sciencedirect.com/science/article/abs/pii/S0378378206001848

4. WHY ELITE ATHLETES MEASURE THEIR CORTISOL

1. Bessel van der Kolk's website https://www.besselvanderkolk.com/
2. A feedback loop is a biological occurrence whereby the output of a system amplifies the system (positive feedback) or inhibits it (negative feedback).

Feedback loops permit living organisms to maintain homeostasis.
3. In a 2021 meta-analysis, several institutions around the world gathered the findings of eight HRV studies. In these cases, participants who monitored their HRV saw clear improvements in certain physiological factors – for instance, lactate threshold – but they saw no statistically meaningful improvement in their cycling or running times. In the end, more research is needed in this space to ensure that athletes are getting the most accurate information possible about their health.
4. The runner, Usain Bolt, makes a bolt sign with his hands before every race. American baseball legend, Barry Bonds, used to kiss the crucifix on his necklace after touching home plate. Fellow baseball great, Sammy Sosa, became famous for his trademark "bunny hop" after every home run.
5. Previous studies have shown contradictory results for non-runner athletes. Weightlifters and rugby players, for example, seemed to benefit from a *rise* in cortisol. Like runners, tennis players and golfers did *not* benefit from a rise in cortisol levels, and for them competition was a severe physiological stressor.
6. https://www.nature.com/articles/s41598-017-06461-z
7. https://www.mdpi.com/2075-1729/11/7/622/htm
8. https://www.nature.com/articles/s41598-017-06461-z
9. https://www.tandfonline.com/doi/abs/10.1080/10615806.2016.1275585

5. STRESS, INFERTILITY, AND CORTISOL

1. "Diagnosis and Treatment of Unexplained Infertility," https://www.ncbi.nlm.nih.gov/pmc/articles/PMC2505167/
2. "Reproductive Problems in Both Men and Women Are Rising at an Alarming Rate," by Shanna H. Swann and Stacey Colino, March 2021, https://www.scientificamerican.com/article/reproductive-problems-in-both-men-and-women-are-rising-at-an-alarming-rate/
3. These modifications were within the guidelines of humane animal treatment.
4. https://www.ncbi.nlm.nih.gov/pmc/articles/PMC3672390/
5. https://academic.oup.com/jcem/article/91/4/1561/2843571.
6. In the general population, 12% of women who try to conceive are diagnosed with infertility.
7. https://ehp.niehs.nih.gov/doi/abs/10.1289/isee.2011.00306
8. "The Effect of Stress on the Semen Quality," https://pubmed.ncbi.nlm.nih.gov/21452563/
9. https://americansforbgu.org/prolonged-stress-can-impact-quality-of-sperm/
10. From a personal conversation with Sarah Berga, MD, May 5, 2022." Percentage calculated from https://academic.oup.com/jcem/article/91/4/1561/2843571
11. https://www.ncbi.nlm.nih.gov/pmc/articles/PMC3672390/
12. https://ajp.psychiatryonline.org/doi/full/10.1176/ajp.155.10.1310
13. https://www.nature.com/articles/3900798

NOTES

6. STRESS, MENOPAUSE, AND CORTISOL

1. For more on allostatic load, see "Allostatic Load and Its Impact on Health: A Systematic Review," https://www.karger.com/Article/FullText/510696#
2. https://www.nature.com/articles/1395453
3. "Reproductive Hormones and the Menopause Transition," https://www.ncbi.nlm.nih.gov/pmc/articles/PMC3197715/
4. "Cortisol Levels During the Menopausal Transition and Early Postmenopause: Observations from the Seattle Midlife Women's Health Study," ncbi.nlm.nih.gov/pmc/articles/PMC2749064/
5. https://journals.lww.com/menopausejournal/Citation/2022/01000/Menopause_symptoms_and_the_cortisol_response.3.aspx
6. https://pubmed.ncbi.nlm.nih.gov/35796211/
7. https://www.debraatkinson.com/
8. https://www.ncbi.nlm.nih.gov/pmc/articles/PMC2749064/

7. WHAT'S THE GUT AND THE MICROBIOME GOT TO DO WITH CORTISOL?

1. As mentioned above, a reciprocal relationship exists between the hypothalamic-pituitary-adrenal (HPA) and the hypothalamic-pituitary-gonadal (HPG) axes wherein the activation of one affects the function of the other and vice versa. See "Stress and the Reproductive Axis," https://www.ncbi.nlm.nih.gov/pmc/articles/PMC4166402/#
2. "Interactions Between Gut Microbiota and Acute Restraint Stress in Peripheral Structures of the Hypothalamic–Pituitary–Adrenal Axis and the Intestine of Male Mice," frontiersin.org/articles/10.3389/fimmu.2019.02655/full
3. https://www.amazon.com/Safe-Uses-Cortisol-William-Jefferies/dp/0398075018
4. from Hans Selye work on General Adaptation Syndrome
5. Microbiome metabolites are produced by bacteria: from dietary components, from host metabolites biochemically modified by gut bacteria, and synthesized de novo by gut microbes.
6. https://pubmed.ncbi.nlm.nih.gov/33503463/#&gid=article-figures%20pid=fig-1-uid-0
7. https://link.springer.com/chapter/10.1007/978-3-030-14358-9_2 - hypothalamic amenorrhea
8. https://www.frontiersin.org/articles/10.3389/fimmu.2017.00598/full
9. https://www.nature.com/articles/s41522-018-0068-z
10. "Western diets, gut dysbiosis, and metabolic diseases: Are they linked?" https://www.ncbi.nlm.nih.gov/pmc/articles/PMC5390820/
11. Ibid.
12. https://www.cell.com/cell/pdf/S0092-8674(21)00754-6.pdf
13. https://www.sciencedirect.com/science/article/pii/S0278584620302670

NOTES

14. https://www.sciencedirect.com/topics/pharmacology-toxicology-and-pharmaceutical-science/irritable-colon
15. https://www.sciencedirect.com/science/article/pii/S0278584620302670#!
16. Also called the "Flemish Gut Flora Project," https://vib.be/flemish-gut-flora-project
17. https://www.science.org/doi/abs/10.1126/science.aad3503

8. CORTISOL AND WEIGHT LOSS: WHY SO MANY DIETS FAIL

1. "Hormone that controls maturation of fat cells discovered," Stanford Medicine, October 25, 2016, https://med.stanford.edu/news/all-news/2016/10/hormone-that-controls-maturation-of-fat-cells-discovered.html
2. *Ibid.*
3. https://www.ncbi.nlm.nih.gov/pmc/articles/PMC4991899/
4. "Impact of Diet in Shaping Gut Microbiota Revealed by a Comparative Study in Children from Europe and Rural Africa," https://www.ncbi.nlm.nih.gov/pmc/articles/PMC2930426/
5. https://pubmed.ncbi.nlm.nih.gov/18421276/
6. https://www.endocrine-abstracts.org/ea/0013/abstracts/poster-presentations/diabetes-metabolism-and-cardiovascular/ea0013p193/
7. Dr. Fung observes that insulin, nonetheless, can still spike due to the release of cortisol, which in turn will stimulate gluconeogenesis – the process of making glucose (sugar) from its own breakdown products or from the breakdown products of lipids (fats) or proteins. This newly made glucose gets released back into the bloodstream where it raises blood glucose levels. Having too much sugar in the blood for long periods of time can cause serious health problems and must be treated.
8. https://pubmed.ncbi.nlm.nih.gov/27861911/
9. Read about Yoshinori Ohsumi, who received the Nobel Prize in Physiology or Medicine (2016) for his investigations into the mechanisms of autophagy. http://www.ohsumilab.aro.iri.titech.ac.jp/english.html
10. https://www.cdc.gov/obesity/data/adult.html
11. "Overweight and Obesity — BMI Statistics." The highest proportions of women considered to be obese were in Estonia (23.6 %), Latvia (25.7 %), Ireland (26.0 %), and Malta (26.7 %). The highest shares of obese men were in Croatia (23.7 %), Ireland (25.7 %), Hungary (25.8 %), and Malta (30.6 %). A higher proportion of men (than women) were pre-obese in each EU Member State. https://ec.europa.eu/eurostat/statistics-explained/index.php?title=Overweight_and_obesity_-_BMI_statistics#Obesity_in_the_EU:_gender_differences
12. "How Stress Makes Us Fat: Cortisol, Diabetes, and Obesity" in The Cortisol Connection by Shawn Talbott, p. 91.
13. "Stress-related Development of Obesity and Cortisol in Women," by Valentina Vicennati, Francesca Pasqui, Carla Cavazza, Uberto Pagotto, and Renato Pasquali, Obesity (2009) 17, 1678–1683, https://www.researchgate.

net/publication/24214176_Stress-related_Development_of_Obesity_and_Cortisol_in_Women
14. Professor Richard J. Johnson talks about "'The Story Behind the Fat Switch," https://www.youtube.com/watch?v=F1afyKN18S0
15. "Relations Between Negative Effect, Coping, and Emotional Eating," https://www.sciencedirect.com/science/article/abs/pii/S0195666306006337
16. Statistics come from the World Health Organization, "Taking Action on Childhood Obesity." https://apps.who.int/iris/bitstream/handle/10665/274792/WHO-NMH-PND-ECHO-18.1-eng.pdf
17. https://pubmed.ncbi.nlm.nih.gov/8549035/

9. CORTISOL FOR THE DIAGNOSIS OF LONG COVID?

1. https://pubmed.ncbi.nlm.nih.gov/26184081/
2. https://www.covid.gov/assets/files/National-Research-Action-Plan-on-Long-COVID-08012022.pdf
3. *Long COVID term was coined by* patients with lingering health problems after SARS-CoV-2 infection
4. Getting to and Sustaining the Next Normal: A Roadmap for Living with COVID (covidroadmap.org)
5. https://www.cdc.gov/nchs/pressroom/nchs_press_releases/2022/20220622.htm
6. Destin Groff, Ashley Sun, Anna E. Ssentongo, Djibril M. Ba, Nicholas Parsons, Govinda R. Poudel, Alain Lekoubou, John S. Oh, Jessica E. Ericson, Paddy Ssentongo, Vernon M. Chinchilli. **Short-term and Long-term Rates of Postacute Sequelae of SARS-CoV-2 Infection: A Systematic Review.** *JAMA Network Open*, 2021; 4 (10): e2128568 DOI: 10.1001/jamanetworkopen.2021.28568
7. https://www.nature.com/articles/s41574-022-00700-8
8. https://www.npr.org/2022/07/31/1114375163/long-covid-longhaulers-disability-labor-ada
9. https://www.mdpi.com/1648-9144/57/10/1087
10. https://www.cell.com/cell/fulltext/S0092-8674(22)00072-1
11. https://www.jstage.jst.go.jp/article/endocrj/advpub/0/advpub_EJ22-0093/_article/-char/ja/
12. https://www.nature.com/articles/s41574-022-00700-8
13. https://www.medrxiv.org/content/10.1101/2022.08.09.22278592v1.full.pdf
14. https://www.bloomberg.com/news/articles/2022-08-11/striking-drop-in-stress-hormone-predicts-long-covid-in-study
15. https://fortune.com/2022/08/12/long-covid-causes-treatment-stress-hormone-cortisol-study/
16. https://www.science.org/content/article/blood-abnormalities-found-people-long-covid
17. https://www.ncbi.nlm.nih.gov/pmc/articles/PMC7163702/

NOTES

18. https://pubmed.ncbi.nlm.nih.gov/12845623/
19. https://pubmed.ncbi.nlm.nih.gov/15488660/
20. https://www.medrxiv.org/content/10.1101/2022.08.09.22278592v1.full.pdf+html
21. https://www.medrxiv.org/content/10.1101/2022.08.09.22278592v1
22. https://www.mdpi.com/1648-9144/57/10/1087/htm
23. https://www.pardigm.com/post/chronic-stress-cortisol-increase-risk-covid-19
24. https://academic.oup.com/jcem/article/106/3/622/6009077
25. https://www.ncbi.nlm.nih.gov/pmc/articles/PMC7368100/
26. https://www.thelancet.com/journals/landia/article/PIIS2213-8587(20)30216-3/fulltext
27. https://jim.bmj.com/content/70/3/766.abstract
28. https://www.mdpi.com/2227-9059/10/7/1527

10. SCIENTIFIC BREAKTHROUGH: MINDSET CONTROLS CORTISOL

1. "Rethinking Stress: The Role of Mindsets in Determining the Stress Response," Alia Crum and Peter Salovey, and Shawn Achor, *Journal of Personality and Social Psychology*, Vol. 104, No. 4, 716–733, 2013.
2. The Austrian psychiatrist Viktor Frankl wrote in *Man's Search for Meaning* that even in a Nazi concentration camp, the inmates who could identify a purpose in life, and who could imagine a positive outcome, had a better chance of surviving camp life than inmates who succumbed to hopelessness.
3. As of 2014, according to the World Health Organization. https://www.who.int/news-room/fact-sheets/detail/diabetes
4. Richard J. Johnson, Professor of Medicine, University of Colorado, has observed that in 1900, diabetes appeared in only 2 of 100,000 people. The same year, obesity affected only 3% of the US population. https://www.youtube.com/watch?v=F1afyKN18S0
5. You can read a summary of Crum and Langer's paper: "Mindset Matters: Exercise and the Placebo Effect," *Psychological Science*, Feb. 18(2):165-71, 2007.
6. To follow more of Alia's groundbreaking work, watch her TEDMED Talk on the power of placebos, or listen to her recent guest spot on the Huberman Lab podcast.

11. RECOMMENDATIONS: HOW TO KEEP YOUR CORTISOL LEVELS BALANCED

1. Perceived Stress Scale proposed by Cohen et al in 1983 - https://www.cmu.edu/dietrich/psychology/stress-immunity-disease-lab/scales/index.html
2. "The effects of aromatherapy on stress and stress responses in adolescents," https://pubmed.ncbi.nlm.nih.gov/19571632/
3. "Acute Effects of Bright Light Exposure on Cortisol Levels," https://www.ncbi.nlm.nih.gov/pmc/articles/PMC3686562/

NOTES

4. "The effect of apple cider vinegar on lipid profiles and glycemic parameters: a systematic review and meta-analysis of randomized clinical trials," https://link.springer.com/article/10.1186/s12906-021-03351-w
5. "Flipping the Metabolic Switch: Understanding and Applying Health Benefits of Fasting," ncbi.nlm.nih.gov/pmc/articles/PMC5783752/
6. "A Review of the Evidence Surrounding the Effects of Breakfast Consumption on Mechanisms of Weight Management," semanticscholar.org/paper/A-Review-of-the-Evidence-Surrounding-the-Effects-of-Gwin-Leidy/10e2ef9e7b8975ad0f43d65e71f2d8c78ab9c3be
7. "High cortisol levels are associated with low quality food choice in type 2 diabetes," https://www.ncbi.nlm.nih.gov/pmc/articles/PMC3253931/
8. Ibid.
9. "Effects of Chronic Social Stress on Obesity," ncbi.nlm.nih.gov/pmc/articles/PMC3428710/
10. "Omega-3 Polyunsaturated Fatty Acid Levels and Dysregulations in Biological Stress Systems," https://pubmed.ncbi.nlm.nih.gov/30077075/
11. https://www.ncbi.nlm.nih.gov/pmc/articles/PMC7520385/
12. "Inadequacy of Immune Health Nutrients: Intakes in US Adults, the 2005–2016 (National Health and Nutrition Examination Surveys)," ncbi.nlm.nih.gov/pmc/articles/PMC7352522/
13. "Scientists Say Vitamin C May Alleviate the Body's Response to Stress,"https://www.sciencedaily.com/releases/1999/08/990823072615.htm
14. "The Effect of 90 Day Administration of a High Dose Vitamin B-complex on Work Stress," https://pubmed.ncbi.nlm.nih.gov/21905094/
15. "B Vitamins and the Brain: Mechanisms, Dose and Efficacy—A Review," ncbi.nlm.nih.gov/pmc/articles/PMC4772032/
16. "Interactions Between Adrenal and Calcium-Regulatory Hormones in Human Health," https://ncbi.nlm.nih.gov/pmc/articles/PMC4123208/
17. "Magnesium deficiency induces anxiety and HPA axis dysregulation: Modulation by therapeutic drug treatment," sciencedirect.com/science/article/pii/S0028390811003054
18. "Superiority of magnesium and vitamin B6 over magnesium alone on severe stress in healthy adults with low magnesemia: A randomized, single-blind clinical trial," https://pubmed.ncbi.nlm.nih.gov/30562392/
19. "Insight into zinc signaling from dietary zinc deficiency," https://www.sciencedirect.com/science/article/abs/pii/S016501730900085X
20. National Institutes of Health, https://ods.od.nih.gov/factsheets/Zinc-HealthProfessional/
21. "Marathon Training and Immune Function," https://pubmed.ncbi.nlm.nih.gov/17465622/
22. "The effects of exercise session timing on weight loss and components of energy balance: midwest exercise trial 2," https://www.nature.com/articles/s41366-019-0409-x#
23. "Plant Adaptogens," https://www.sciencedirect.com/science/article/abs/pii/S0944711311800255
24. "A Prospective, Randomized Double-Blind, Placebo-Controlled Study of Safety and Efficacy of a High-Concentration Full-Spectrum Extract of

NOTES

Ashwagandha Root in Reducing Stress and Anxiety in Adults," https://www.ncbi.nlm.nih.gov/pmc/articles/PMC3573577/

25. "Rosenroot (Rhodiola rosea): Traditional use, chemical composition, pharmacology and clinical efficacy," sciencedirect.com/science/article/abs/pii/S094471131000036X
26. *Ibid.*
27. *Ibid.*
28. "Efficacy and Safety of Ginseng," https://nutradvance.pt/wp-content/uploads/2016/04/Ref56.download1.php_.pdf
29. "Effect of Magnolia officinalis and Phellodendron amurense (Relora®) on cortisol and psychological mood state in moderately stressed subjects,"https://ncbi.nlm.nih.gov/pmc/articles/PMC3750820/
30. "Metabolic flexibility in health and disease," https://ncbi.nlm.nih.gov/pmc/articles/PMC5513193/
31. "Mindsets: Q&A with Dr. Alia Crum, Stanford Psychology," https://www.parulsomani.com/post/mindsets-q-a-with-dr-alia-crum-stanford-psychology
32. "Dr. Alia Crum: Science of Mindsets for Health & Performance | Huberman Lab Podcast #56," https://www.youtube.com/watch?v=dFR_wFN23ZY
33. https://pubmed.ncbi.nlm.nih.gov/32819304/
34. See "Cold Showers, Hot Saunas and the New Way to Tame Stress," by Betsy Morris, https://www.wsj.com/articles/what-is-hormetic-stress-and-how-does-it-work-11647179278
35. Women's response to stress may more frequently be "tend and befriend." See Biobehavioral Responses to Stress in Females: Tend-and-Befriend, Not Fight-or-Flight, https://taylorlab.psych.ucla.edu/wp-content/uploads/sites/5/2014/10/2000_Biobehavioral-responses-to-stress-in-females_tend-and-befriend.pdf
36. https://www.ncbi.nlm.nih.gov/pmc/articles/PMC7520385/
37. "Repeated exposure with short-term behavioral stress resolves pre-existing stress-induced depressive-like behavior in mice," nature.com/articles/s41467-021-26968-4
38. "The geroscience agenda: Toxic stress, hormetic stress, and the rate of aging," https://www.ncbi.nlm.nih.gov/pmc/articles/PMC7520385/
39. https://pubmed.ncbi.nlm.nih.gov/32979553/
40. https://giving.ucsf.edu/stories/exploring-stress-paradox-prevent-disease
41. "Preconditioning in neuroprotection: From hypoxia to ischemia," https://www.ncbi.nlm.nih.gov/pmc/articles/PMC5515698/
42. "Association Between Sauna Bathing and Fatal Cardiovascular and All-Cause Mortality Events," https://jamanetwork.com/journals/jamainternalmedicine/fullarticle/2130724
43. https://www.ncbi.nlm.nih.gov/pmc/articles/PMC4034215/
44. https://pubmed.ncbi.nlm.nih.gov/34175558/
45. https://pubmed.ncbi.nlm.nih.gov/33716913/
46. https://www.sciencedirect.com/science/article/pii/S0306987718305723#b1085
47. https://pubmed.ncbi.nlm.nih.gov/26135345/
48. https://pubmed.ncbi.nlm.nih.gov/28115234/
49. https://pubmed.ncbi.nlm.nih.gov/31060881/

NOTES

50. https://www.intechopen.com/chapters/57745
51. https://med.stanford.edu/stresshealthcenter.html
52. https://hypnotechs.com/resources/spiegel-test/ by psychiatrist Herbert Spiegel, who was the father of David Spiegel and a specialist in hypnosis

PARDIGM.COM INTRO

1. Check which latest models are supported.

Made in the USA
Las Vegas, NV
01 November 2023